Primal Moms Look Good Naked

A MOTHER'S GUIDE TO ACHIEVING BEAUTY THROUGH EXCELLENT HEALTH

Victory Belt Publishing Inc.

Las Vegas

First Published in 2013 by Victory Belt Publishing Inc.

Copyright © 2013 Peggy Emch

ISBN 13: 978-1-936608-66-9

The information included in this book is for educational purposes only. It is not intended nor implied to be a substitute for professional medical advice. The reader should always consult his or her healthcare provider to determine the appropriateness of the information for their own situation or if they have any questions regarding a medical condition or treatment plan. Reading the information in this book does not create a physician-patient relationship.

Printed in the USA
RRD 01-13

Exercise photo credit, Julian Mondragon.

Contents

The research for this book is dedicated to my late sister Liz

Acknowledgments

With deep appreciation I would like to thank my husband, Julian, for helping me make time for the writing of this book and listening to me bounce ideas around day and night. I would like to thank my daughter, Evelyn, for kindly giving me room to think. And I would like to apologize to Maya for growing inside my belly with maybe a little more stress than was ideal. I would also like to thank her for appearing in the middle of this project. Being pregnant while writing a book on pregnancy was an unexpected advantage. I am also grateful to my publisher, Victory Belt, for allowing me creative liberty and independence, and for offering the hand of such incredible editors and illustrators. I will forever thank my sister for being such an inspiration to explore and question conventional thinking. Thank you Ryan and Kristy for your help on Tuesday. And last, these acknowledgements would not be complete without thanking my readers for their support and encouragement.

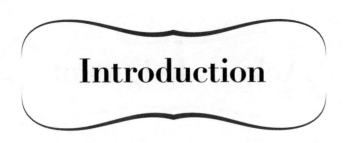

Introduction

The idea that a mother can look good naked might seem crazy to you, especially if you and any mom you've ever known bears the unflattering scars of pregnancy. Sure, there are a lucky few who seem to miraculously make it through unscathed, but for most of us, looking good without clothes after having a baby or two is a dream, right? Well, what if it doesn't have to be? What if there is a way to keep the physical changes of pregnancy and birth from marring your body?

You might find this hard to believe. Or maybe, like me, you feel that our bodies are actually astonishingly resilient, and having a baby should not be a sacrifice of beauty and body function

Just think about it. Why should pregnancy leave women hopelessly overweight, scarred with stretch marks and bulging varicose veins? Why should it leave us suffering from incontinence, or in need of corsets and cinchers to hold in sagging skin and bulging bellies? None of this makes any functional sense! Why would nature have failed women so profoundly? Can it really be that after hundreds of thousands of years on earth and billions of babies born, women's bodies haven't evolved to handle the stretch of the expanding belly or the increased flow of blood?

In fact, nature did not fail us. We failed ourselves when we moved away from a simpler way of life. You can easily find examples of nature's fine design in women living traditional hunter-gatherer lifestyles, where food isn't intended to last until after your death, where it is pulled from the ground rather than packaged in plastic bags, cans, or boxes. In these cultures, you'll find mothers with smooth, supple skin, free of cellulite and varicose veins, whose bodies look as healthy and strong as they did before they conceived children.

Am I romanticizing here? No. And I speak from experience. Before I got pregnant with my first child, I adopted a Primal diet and lifestyle to help alleviate chronic health issues, one of which was infertility. This way of eating and exercising was so healing that my fertility quickly returned and I found myself unexpectedly pregnant. Furthermore, and despite my previous health problems, I escaped the countless discomforts women experience both during and after pregnancy. I expected that since I had suffered most of my life from joint and skin problems, from depression and hormonal imbalances, and both low and high blood sugar, I would have been high risk for many associated pregnancy complications. In fact, I didn't get stretch marks or varicose veins or postpartum depression or preeclampsia or morning sickness; breastfeeding was easy, I was happy and healthy, and my daughter, Evelyn, was beautiful in every way. On top of all that, I maintained my fitness and was soon back to my pre-pregnancy weight.

What made my experience so different from that of other modern women? This question stayed with me for many years and prompted the research that led to this book. I have learned that our bodies were actually designed to be strong and resilient, and that when they aren't it is simply because they are out of balance. In the following pages, I will present evidence that the female body is perfectly capable of bearing children without being compromised in the process. I will show that women don't have to suffer depression and fatigue, or give up shorts and bathing suits after the birth of a child.

In *Primal Moms Look Good Naked,* I focus on how a mother's body looks for two reasons. First, because we are humans, and humans like to look good. This is not pure vanity; according to Darwin and other evolutionary theorists, we want to be attractive so that we can, yes, attract mates and reproduce. Second, and more importantly, we want to look good because beauty (clear eyes, firm skin, strong muscles, etc.) is a direct reflection of health. When our bodies are healthy, they are *naturally* attractive; when there are malformations, the attractiveness diminishes. And as you will soon see, the traits we typically consider unattractive are caused by malnutrition, inflammation, and imbalanced hormones, among other things. Beauty is far less random than we have been led to believe.

The advice I impart in this book will make you look and feel better than you ever did before you got pregnant. Best of all, you will pass this health on to your baby so that he or she is born with all the advantages that health brings, including stronger minds and bodies. You can do all this by simply trading some aspects of your modern lifestyle for a Primal one.

PART I

The Wisdom of Our Ancestors

Good nutrition, which can usually prevent early physical degeneration, is something we can learn from our ancient ancestors and those currently living lives untouched by civilization. Those who have existed in unity with the earth for thousands of years have a keen, intuitive awareness of what the body needs and how and where to get the materials to make it strong.

The lives of ancient peoples revolved around very basic needs: finding and preparing food and shelter, fertility, and community. This is in contrast to our own lives, where food is generally an afterthought and chosen for convenience rather than nutrition. Our food is processed by big corporations, and we have therefore given them the power to choose what we put in our bodies. We have stopped paying attention to what we put in our mouths to focus on other things, like the progress of civilization—an arguably noble cause for mankind but a destructive one for our bodies. Health and healing used to be things we were responsible for, but with the advancement of science and technology we have passed that responsibility on to other people. Instead of taking care of the one body which we will have until we die, we let doctors tell us what to do; when it degenerates, we turn to medication to patch it up. Clearly, this isn't working out too well.

Modern medicine has proven its value in surgery and emergency procedures, but it falls short in healing chronic illness—the biggest killer of modern man. For that we must rely on nutrition. The nutrition I speak of isn't the familiar modern dietary science that has given us low fat diets, high protein diets, zero-carb diets, vegetarian and vegan diets, raw diets, the alkaline diet, or super food diets. While there are threads of value running through each of these diet plans, I am talking about the nutrition developed through centuries of natives living in accordance with nature, who depend on robust health for their survival. These people do not suffer from chronic disease because centuries of gathered wisdom has taught them how to be strong and resilient. These are the people we should seek out to answer our questions about health and nutrition.

When we want to fix our cars, we go to a car repairman, not a gardener. When we need our taxes done, we go to a tax specialist, not a baker. When we want a house built, we go to a carpenter, not a philosopher. Likewise, when we want good health, we shouldn't visit a chemist, we should look for answers from an expert—someone with a family line that is strong, robust, and healthy, and who has avoided illness by carefully selecting nourishing foods. Our ancestors didn't spend their time memorizing presidents or solving mathematical problems. They observed the earth and what it has to offer us. They observed their bodies and the animals and plants around them. And they drew conclusions about these observations. These are not the people who have seen a 600 percent increase in autism within the last three decades, and an over 60 percent increase in diabetes, and over 70 percent increase in obesity in the last decade. When it comes to health, we are not the experts. It is time we start learning from those who are.

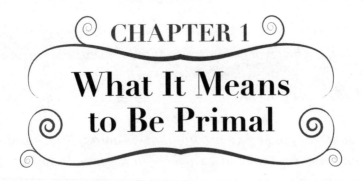

CHAPTER 1

What It Means to Be Primal

Primal and Paleo are words that are used to refer to a primitive way of eating that can be adopted by modern people. They have become buzzwords much like the words vegan and low-carb. The Paleo diet is often attacked as a fad—a diet that doesn't offer any real benefit to the body and is simply a food trend or form of rebellion. But the ideas behind Paleo and Primal are much more than that. The health differences between hunter-gatherers and agriculturists have been well documented in present day tribes and in fossil artifacts. What's behind the fascination with Primal and Paleo lifestyles is a recognition of what's wrong with our food supply, our lifestyle, and how it affects our bodies. The central ideas of both emphasize what works best for human physiology.

Primal or Paleo?

When I first went "Paleo" in 2005, it had a pretty strict definition. As defined by Dr. Loren Cordain, the founder of The Paleo Diet, it includes wild meats, fruits, and veggies, and excludes just about everything processed. It is simple. It is healing. And it is generally very successful. The Primal diet was first popularized by Aajonus Vonderplanitz, who advocates eating a raw, primarily carnivorous, diet. His diet includes raw vegetable juices and raw animal foods, including raw milk; he has been using his Primal diet to heal very sick people for the last 35 years. Mark Sisson, author of *The Primal Blueprint*, made the Primal-type diet more practical for 21st century living by allowing the meat and vegetables to be cooked, and allowing for 100 grams of carbs plus 20 percent room for error. At this point, there are at least 20 different approaches to eating optimally in a Primal or Paleo manner. Each of them is influenced by its founder's personal health history, along with science and traditional wisdom.

Over the years, I have tried many versions of Paleo, Primal, traditional, and hunter-gatherer diets—more than was in any way convenient. However, as a result of my flexibility, I have healed longstanding health issues and learned a valuable lesson: There are infinite ways to be Primal. Because of differences in climate, the availability of specific plants and animals, the proximity of other tribes with which to trade, the time of year, the period in history, and the geography of the land, the diets of our Primal ancestors varied dramatically. There is no one way to be Primal just as there is no one optimal Primal diet.

I prefer the word Primal over Paleo because Paleo implies a time in history, the Paleolithic Era, and what was available then. For me, Primal emphasizes a spirit and a way of living that is natural, dynamic, and harmonious. Hence, Paleo allows for all kinds of treats as long as each ingredient is "legal," while Primal tries to keep in line with how people might have lived and ate. You simply can't be Primal (optimally healthy and, arguably, truly human) if you don't get sunshine and fresh air, if you don't experience nature, pull and push heavy things, run, jump, eat the whole animal (even if the only animals you eat are fish). But it doesn't require that you eat beef or bacon; you don't have to eat meat at all. Being a modern Primal human means that you make an effort to think, to live, and to eat in ways that mimic our ancestors.

The Paleolithic Period and Evolution

The Paleolithic period extended throughout most of human history—i.e., from the time of the earliest discovered tools, around 2.6 million years ago, until the time when agriculture began to replace hunting and gathering, around 10 thousand years ago. We think the dietary habits of these ancient ancestors are important from an evolutionary perspective because evolution works so incredibly slowly. Our bodies have not evolved much at all in the last 10,000 years because evolution, in most cases, takes many tens of thousands of years to affect noticeable change. In short, our bodies have not adapted to the consumption of potato chips and soda over the last 50 years, the lack of omega 3s in the diet, or the sedentary lifestyles of the 20th century. We've got about 20,000 years to go before we actually adapt to the couch potato lifestyle.

While we can only speculate about the specifics of Paleolithic diet and lifestyle, we can use the real observations of modern hunter-gatherers and the archaeological remains of ancient hunter-gatherers to draw conclusions about activities and food and their effects on health. Some hunter-gatherers ate a lot of starch, some more recent animal herders, like Africa's Masai, eat fermented dairy. People who lived in northern climates ate less plant matter and more meat; coastal hunter-gatherers ate lots of seafood. Humans have thrived on a variety of diets and for this reason there is no "original human diet," and there doesn't need to be. Katherine Milton of the University of

California, Berkeley, who studies the dietary ecology of primates, including ancient and modern humans, agrees with this point of view. In her article, "Hunter-Gatherer Diets—A Different Perspective," she notes:

Data on modern-day hunter-gatherers as well as hunter-gatherer-agriculturalists who consume traditional diets indicate that such societies are largely free of diseases of civilization regardless of whether a high percentage of dietary energy is supplied by wild animal foods (e.g., in Canadian Eskimos), wild plant foods (e.g., in the !Kung), or domesticated plant foods taken primarily from a single cultivar (e.g., in the Yanomamo)."

Which approach works best for an individual? That will vary. To begin to figure out the right types of food for you, begin by eliminating grains, legumes, sugar, and other modern processed foods. Then listen to your body for signs of imbalance, and adjust the macronutrient (carbs, fats, and protein) ratios according to your activity level, genetics, health conditions, and so forth. Don't worry, I will detail how to do this later in the book.

Hunter-Gatherers

The practices of hunter-gatherers, unlike those of our own culture, are in tune with the natural world. According to researchers and Westerners who have spent significant time interacting with hunter-gatherers, these men and women are largely free of the symptoms of malnutrition, which too many people suffer from here in the US. You can get an idea for how beautiful hunter-gatherer women remain after pregnancy and into old age without even leaving your home. Simply watch documentaries like IMAX's *Amazon*, National Geographic's *Gun, Germs and Steel*, The BBC's *Tribe* (viewed on the Discovery Channel as *Going Tribal in the US*), and the Travel Channel's *Mark and Ollie: Living With the Tribes*. Their teeth are straight, their hair is thick into old age, and they are free of cellulite and stretch marks.

Hunter-gatherers never eat Funyuns or Snickers bars. They haven't had foods fried in refined vegetable oil—a substance which not only does not exist in nature, but which is produced in ways that make it hard for our bodies to process. They don't eat whole grains and, if they did, they would remove the toxins by eating them freshly ground and fermented. They don't have the machines used for processing cereal, the modern staple which we drown in milk first burned by pasteurization (and, worse, ultra-pasteurization) and then passed through sieves with microscopic holes, reducing the size of the fat molecules and preventing them from floating to the top (all that so it will *look more appetizing*). They've never drunk the dark fizzy cola that leaches calcium from bones, and they've never eaten a cow whose flesh is acidic from eating grains it wasn't designed to digest. Our pantries are filled with a labyrinth of boxed and canned foods that have been scientifically modified with the sole purpose of addicting us to new flavors and textures. The "pantries" of hunter-gatherers are the small pouches they carry, filled with fresh foods pulled from rich soil.

Hunter-gatherer's eat simple foods and lead simpler lives that are in harmony with the earth. They don't have to navigate rush hour traffic or worry about deadlines or mortgages or paying for a child's college education. They don't have a lot of material possessions that need to be replaced or fixed. They have worries, mostly about natural dangers, but they don't live with the daily stresses that occur in modern life.

Stress

One of the challenges of modern life, even for a Primal-minded person, is keeping stress levels low. And in order to achieve optimum health and beauty, we *must* make stress-management a priority.

Many of the symptoms from which most of us commonly suffer—e.g., headaches, muscle spasms, hair loss, mouth ulcers, reproductive problems, skin problems—can be caused by excessive, chronic stress. The adrenal glands are responsible for managing stress in our bodies. These glands produce cortisol and adrenaline, the hormones which the body uses to protect itself. When stress becomes very high over extended periods of time, the adrenals overwork and eventually become depleted. Once this happens, it will be very difficult to manage stress at all.

According to Dr. Barry Sears, "if you are overproducing corticosteroids, especially cortisol, you will bring all eicosanoid [prostaglandin] synthesis to a crashing halt—including the shut-down of the immune system."

All of these symptoms are linked to nutritional deficiencies and hormonal imbalances, but often stress is the underlying cause of those deficits. Too much stress during childhood, due to, say, abuse or abandonment, can lead to a lifetime of health problems. Car accidents or sports accidents can turn a once healthy person into a physical mess. Long-term marital issues can lead to severe depression, back pain, and other health conditions.

Unfortunately, in today's world, these problems are all too common. But it's not just big trauma that causes stress. There are the everyday agitations of incessantly barking dogs, chronically sick or hyper children, loud noises, traffic, schedule demands, contentious interactions with people, illness, and financial difficulties. And there is the stress caused (and exacerbated) by the nutrient deficiencies inherent in eating irresponsibly.

Examples of physical stressors:

+ Colds, flus, allergies
+ Falling and bumping into things
+ Chronic pain like arthritis or carpal tunnel syndrome
+ Toxic overload from food
+ Toxic overload from pollution in water and air
+ Malnutrition

Examples of psychological stressors:

+ Fights with spouse or children
+ Death of a loved one
+ Perfectionism and insecurity
+ Pressures at work and school
+ Schedule demands
+ Financial troubles
+ Broken down cars and household things
+ Sudden loud noises

Examples of nutritional stressors:

+ Magnesium, which is important for many body processes, gets quickly depleted during chronic or acute high stress. Even loud noises—like a car crash or a rock concert—can lower magnesium levels.
+ Omega-3 fatty acid deficiency, which is very common, prohibits the body from producing good prostaglandins. Good prostaglandins are anti-inflammatory and enhance immune health. They are so important that, without them, a person can end up with high blood pressure, heart attacks, and arthritis. Cortisol—the stress hormone—also stands in the way of good prostaglandin production.

Managing stress

For most of us, eliminating stress completely is not an option. We can't change the personalities of our loved ones, we do not have control over our spouse's words and actions, we may not know what is wrong with our children, we may not have the money to fix our cars. But improving our nutrition is something we *can* do. Eschewing junk food is an option. I have found, as have many others, that improved nutrition is an excellent first step towards eliminating stress. The problems are still there, but how we react to them begins to change. And stress is all about reactions.

Lifestyle

Of course, we are not completely powerless to stress. We can reduce stress by simplifying our lives. How many kitchen utensils do you really *need*? Is that $3,000 set of nursery furniture really necessary when your monthly income barely pays the bills? Must your kids have all those toys, and do you actually need every new gadget that hits the market? How about the expensive cars, the mortgage you can barely afford, and all the things we own that break and must be replaced? Is all of the *stuff* really necessary?

As I said, choosing a simpler diet is your best first step. But from there, you can begin to think about a major shift in lifestyle. The main concerns of our ancestors were food, safety, and community. Their lives revolved around nature and people, not things. For us, being Primal will never be quite so simple, but it can be *simpler*. Lowering the strain on our bodies and our minds is what modern Primal living is all about.

Years ago, before I started thinking about these things, I was living the typical stressed out American life. I lived in the San Francisco Bay Area and worked at a job I hated so that I could afford expensive day care for my daughter. I drove home every day in rush hour traffic in a car I couldn't afford. I continually worried that my boss might fire me. I had no family nearby to support me. I borrowed money and wondered how I would ever pay it back. My life was not Primal, but since I ate Primal-type foods I thought I was on the right track. But I was still stressed. Once I understood the lifestyle link to being Primal, things got so much easier. I moved to a city where I could ride my bike everywhere I needed to go. I sold my car, reduced my expenses, and stopped borrowing money. I shifted my focus to my hobbies, my family, and the natural world around me. Big changes like these aren't easy to make and it takes time to implement them. We stumble along the way, but it is worth it for ourselves and our children.

New parents are even more susceptible to the stress of material things. New moms are pressured from all directions into buying a hundred unnecessary items for their babies. In reality, they need very little. When I was pregnant the first time, I didn't even have a TV, but I thought I had to buy everything in Babies"R"Us (which is just embarrassing to think of now). I was brainwashed! I have a second baby on the way, and, thankfully, buying stuff is very low on my list of priorities. I'll need a few things, but not much.

Without all of the things to purchase, to set up and fumble with, to plan, and to maintain, raising a baby is actually pretty relaxing and easy. They are remarkably simple creatures: they sleep most of the time, and are perfectly happy just to be in your arms and go where you go. They require little more than a nipple, soft voices, and a loving embrace. We are so programmed to overschedule ourselves and our children, but if you're not running all over town every day, trying to keep up with a busy, modern life, there's actually plenty to take care of yourself, to plan a clean diet, and to exercise (especially if you keep your baby close to you in a sling).

CHAPTER 2

My Story:
PCOS, Celiac, and a New Beginning

By now you are probably wondering what gives me the right to tell you how to eat and live. I am not an MD or a nutritionist but, rather, a once unhealthy, now vigorous woman who has a passion for learning and sharing. I experienced many of the conditions I write about in this book long before I became pregnant. I visited MDs for help with everything from infertility, to weak joints, to depression. Their medicines, tests, and procedures failed me, and so I began researching their causes myself. I have since learned a great deal about how to prevent and repair the conditions that plague pregnant and postpartum women. I write about health and nutrition because doctors are more interested in covering up symptoms than in giving us ways to truly heal. I want to offer women hope and the tools they need to feel and look as healthy as possible.

Polycystic Ovarian Syndrome (PCOS)

I started menstruating too young—I was barely eleven—and my cycles were irregular. All of my adult life I had amenorrhea (infrequent periods), which was not caused by being underweight or overactive but by not having enough progesterone (making it impossible for the egg to move out of the ovaries). But from the beginning, when my periods did come, they were heavy and excruciatingly painful. When the body doesn't produce enough progesterone, cysts form, and when those cysts rupture the pain is inexplicable. In addition, I was moody, pimply, and depressed. You've heard of PMS, or maybe you suffer from it yourself? Well, take that and put it on steroids and you'll understand PCOS. Getting my period so young forced me to grow up too soon, and I was in no way prepared for the pain and confusion of imbalanced hormones.

Around 5 million women (**one in 15** in the US) have PCOS, a masculinizing hormonal imbalance. In women with PCOS, the ovaries produce an excess of male hormones (androgens), making it difficult or impossible for the ovaries to release an egg. This leads to cysts on the ovaries and a host of troublesome symptoms.

Symptoms of PCOS:

+ Irregular or absent periods
+ Pelvic pain
+ Cysts on the ovaries
+ Infertility
+ Depression
+ Acne
+ Weight gain
+ Hair loss and facial hair growth (hirsutism)
+ Sleep apnea

The Cause of PCOS

While there are many factors such as obesity, genetics, and exposure to synthetic estrogens that can predispose a woman to PCOS, the root cause is insulin resistance.

Insulin is what our bodies use to regulate blood glucose, which must be kept within a specific range at all times. The pancreas produces insulin to help glucose pass through the cell walls so that it can be used for energy. Insulin resistance arises when blood sugar levels are elevated long-term and the pancreas overproduces insulin to keep the blood sugar levels within a healthy range. After years of this abuse, the cells become desensitized to insulin and blood sugar regulation is impaired. At this point, the blood sugar will remain high and the body can do nothing to bring it down to a healthy level. This same problem leads to diabetes. For women, PCOS is often the first stop on the road to diabetes.

Excess insulin floating around the bloodstream wreaks havoc on the body in many ways. As it relates to PCOS, free-floating insulin stimulates the ovaries to produce excess testosterone, which, as mentioned above, prevents the ovaries from releasing an egg each month—a *leading cause of infertility*. (When cells become resistant to insulin, the glucose must make its way to the liver to be converted to fat instead of being used as energy by the cells. This is why women suffering from PCOS are often overweight.)

Insulin resistance can come about through eating a diet high in refined carbohydrates and low in nutrients. Other factors that contribute to hormonal imbalances such as PCOS are exposure to pollution, plastics, other chemicals, and the synthetic hormones found in conventional beef. These synthetic compounds contain xenoestrogens (synthetic or environmental estrogens). These environmental estrogens disrupt our delicate hormonal system by mimicking real estrogen. The body responds by producing excessive amounts of other hormones in an attempt to balance the estrogen.

Once the body's hormones become imbalanced, symptoms start surfacing. The hair loss, acne, and dark facial hair growth didn't start for me until my twenties, but debilitating menstruation, cysts, and depression were there from the beginning. In a way, my young body was getting old. While I should have been a carefree kid, I was depressed, shy, and in pain.

I pushed on despite my health problems, as most of us do, and found solace in learning and exercise. I hiked. I ran long distances. I learned to snowboard. I got bachelor's degrees in mathematics and philosophy and taught myself basic Spanish and how to play the piano and to sing. I read about everything under the sun—including lots of books on health science. I started taking an interest in nutrition and made friends with other health-minded folk. One day, in 2003, one of them casually suggested that she might know the cause of my persistent stomachaches. Little did I know that, as a result of our conversation, my life was about to change forever.

Celiac Disease

Celiac disease is a disorder of the immune system—an autoimmune disease. This means that the immune system essentially mounts an attack on its own body. In the case of celiac disease, the attack is on the lining of the small intestine. The small intestine has a lining of tiny, hair-like villi that absorb nutrients. In celiacs, these villi become paralyzed, impairing the absorption of certain nutrients. In time, this causes severe nutritional deficiencies, and in children it can be the cause of failure to thrive. Adult celiacs usually have really weird things going on with their digestion, like bloating, diarrhea, gas, distention, plus all kinds of other difficulties you wouldn't want to witness. But the digestive problems are just the tip of the iceberg. Gluten—the protein found in wheat, rye, and barley which celiacs react to—can be responsible for schizophrenia, depression, paranoia, ADD, joint and bone problems, myopia (near sightedness), hormonal problems, poor wound healing and other skin problems (from zinc deficiency)—the list goes on. Humans need nutrients to survive and to thrive. Without them, the body makes sacrifices to save the vital organs while other systems suffer. The life of an undiagnosed celiac is often very difficult, both emotionally and physically, and it is also often shorter than average.

Needless to say, I was eager to try a gluten-free diet after my friend described the symptoms. I had never heard of autoimmune disorders but, at this point, my digestion was so messed up that I would have tried anything to fix it. Immediately after eliminating gluten from my diet, many things started to change. My joints—which had been slipping out of their sockets since I was eleven—stayed put. My eyesight, which had been getting progressively worse since childhood (I was nearing legal blindness by the time I was 26), stopped degenerating from that day forward. My depression started to ease up, my periods became regular and painless, and, after an entire adult life of infertility, I got pregnant.

My body began to work better in every way the moment it started getting nutrients. But of course, what takes two decades to destroy takes time to repair. Ideally, I would have waited a long time to have a baby in order to build my nutrient stores. My body had been severely malnourished for many years. It doesn't just take a few months to reverse that. But I had no way of knowing at the time that changing my diet would change my fertility. No doctor had mentioned this connection so, after years of not using birth control, I was pregnant—ready or not.

My First Primal Pregnancy

There were no guides on any of this back then and, even now, there are only a few. When I made the transition in 2005, I read two books about the Paleo diet: Dr. Loren Cordain's *The Paleo Diet* and Ray Audette's *Neanderthin*. Those two books, in addition to my love of nature, were enough to make me feel confident about eating Primally, even while pregnant. At this point I had little regard for conventional methods. I was happy to venture out on my own with my baby. Living in accordance with nature couldn't possibly hurt me as much as the American diet and medical system already had. I explained this to my friends and family and the plan was generally well received. I got lucky with my obstetrician. He was Japanese and had no problem with a diet free of "healthy whole grains," dairy, and heart healthy vegetable oils. His wife hadn't eaten those foods herself while pregnant. We both knew I couldn't do my baby any harm by eating a variety of fruits, nuts, meats, roots, tubers, and vegetables.

I had always been grounded by my love of nature. I understood that packaged food was not ideal human food, that a hectic lifestyle was not healthy, that nature is important, and that strong communities make strong individuals. But there were many preconceptions about which I remained totally clueless. For example, I still thought that pregnant women had to get fat and always got stretch marks. I was pretty sure I could say goodbye to my six pack. I had no reason to believe that any pregnant woman could be even-tempered. I expected to be miserable and unattractive by the end of those nine months. But as the months went by, I was amazed when *none* of those things happened. Obviously I still had a lot to learn about what is natural and what is not. What I began to realize was that the problems common during pregnancy are the result of deviating from natural ways."

This would be my journey for the next several years: to learn what it really means to be a member of the animal kingdom and not some industrial imposter. While I was pregnant and in the years that followed, I was strict about eating a diet of nothing but Primal foods. I was devoted to learning about the diets of primitive people and the ways in which they raised their children. Diet was a key element, but so was the method of child rearing. I held my baby constantly, carried her in a sling, sung to her often, used cloth diapers, breast fed for one-and-a-half years, and didn't over-sterilize her environment. I studied how to live *naturally,* and as a result I have been rewarded with a remarkably happy, gifted, beautiful child. Sure, there is probably some amount of luck involved, and maybe a little bit of good genetics, but over all she and I are doing better than I could have ever dreamed—at least based on all the examples around me.

CHAPTER 3

Fertility, Conception, and Child Spacing

Infertility is a big problem in modern culture. According to the Centers for Disease Control and Prevention (CDC), 10 percent (6.1 million) of women are infertile. Of course, the numbers are probably much higher. Infertility in women who are uninsured or never seek help goes unreported. Many of these cases are avoidable and reversible through some simple changes in diet and the addition of certain nutrients.

The same problems of fertility can be seen in other animal species when they are taken off of their traditional diets. Francis M. Pottenger researched this phenomenon extensively in the 1930s with cats. He observed, throughout a ten-year research project, that cats given anything other than a raw carnivorous diet suffer degeneration and pass down these defects to their offspring, making each subsequent generation weaker and weaker. Dr. Pottenger proved that the type and quality of food eaten during pregnancy is critical for good bone structure and reproductive health. In his study, he had two groups of cats, those that ate raw meats and raw milk and those that ate cooked meats and pasteurized milk. The cats in the cooked meat and milk group produced cats with infertility and birth defects in the next generation. The cats in the raw meat and milk group consistently produced robust and fertile cats. Zookeepers also realize that deviating too far from an animal's native diet can lead to symptoms of disease. Scientists routinely induce modern disease in lab rats by altering their diets. Researchers have observed this phenomenon among humans who have been "civilized" or pulled out of their natural environment. One such example is the Inuit Eskimos. Traditionally, their diet consisted mainly of whale, walrus, seal, caribou, and fish, plus small amounts of local tubers, berries, and seaweed. They had eaten this way for many thousands of years and it had served them well. When they were resettled in towns and began eating wheat and other modern, refined foods, they were suffering from previously unknown diseases within two generations.

Fertility Nutrients

Certain nutrients are necessary for fertility. Without them a woman will have no luck getting pregnant. Many of us are deficient in one or more of these essential nutrients without even realizing it. A woman may suffer from eczema, for example, and have no idea that it might be related to her infertility; Vitamin A deficiency can underlie both conditions. Or a woman with severe symptoms of PMS may have no idea that it's linked to the same Vitamin D deficiency that is also causing her infertility.

Folate, iodine, iron, Vitamins A, D, E, K2, B12, iodine, zinc, and adequate fat and protein are all necessary for fertility. Of course, there are many more nutrients required to grow a healthy baby, but these are the nutrients which, when absent, might prevent conception. Consider, too, that the phytic acid in grains, legumes, and nuts prevents the absorption of many of these nutrients. Thus, what we *don't* eat may have as much of an influence on fertility as what we do eat.

Foods which have been traditionally considered essential for fertility and pregnancy are raw dairy from cows grazing on green grass, organs such as liver, heart, and kidney, as well as egg yolks, seafood, and leafy greens. The following are some specific nutrients that help to prevent and correct infertility issues.

- **Vitamin D** plays a role in the maturation and growth of the egg follicle. It is needed to make sex hormones, and it acts with estrogen to prepare a sufficient lining for the uterus. Vitamin D can be obtained from cod liver oil, organ meats, wild salmon, and sunlight.

- **Vitamin A** promotes better sperm-nourishing cervical fluid. Low Vitamin A can reduce the fluid which sperm need to swim through to meet the egg. In its true form, Vitamin A can only be obtained from animal sources. Plant Vitamin A, or beta-carotene, can be obtained from plants but must be combined with fats in order for the liver to produce the bile salts necessary for absorption. Vitamin A is found in high concentrations in butter from grass-fed cows, fish eggs, wild salmon, and liver.

- **Vitamin K2** is a lesser-known vitamin required for both bone growth and fertility. It is found in liver, shellfish, organ meats, butter from grass-fed cows, and fermented foods such as sauerkraut and natto (fermented soybeans).

- **Vitamin E** is important in all stages of pregnancy and even helps prevent miscarriage. Since there are approximately 100 isomers of Vitamin E in foods and only 16 are added to the most expensive supplements (with only one or two being added to the cheapest), it is best to focus on obtaining it from foods. Vitamin E can be found in olive oil, avocadoes, green leafy vegetables, and almonds.

- **Fats** are critical in ample amounts in the diet because they carry fat-soluble vitamins—Vitamins A, D, K2, and E. Without sufficient fat in the diet, we can't use the fat-soluble vitamins, no matter how much we eat. Fat should *never* be restricted in your diet if you are pregnant or trying to conceive.

- **Vitamin B6** balances estrogen and progesterone. A lack of it is associated with infertility. It can be found in raw milk, leafy green salads, seared and raw tuna, and banana. Vitamin B6 is heat sensitive and therefore diminishes when cooked.

- **Vitamin B12** has been shown to aid conception in anemic women. This essential nutrient can only be obtained from animal products because the body can't make it by itself. Just about any animal food contains it. However, it's not readily absorbed in people with impaired digestion, hence most of us, and not just vegetarians, are deficient in B12.

- **Folate** (not the synthetic folic acid variant found in most vitamin supplements) is necessary for conception to even take place. It also prevents the horrible disease spina bifida, which is characterized by devastating brain and spinal cord defects. Liver, leafy greens, nuts, and chicken all contain folate, with chicken liver being the richest source.

- **Zinc** is also required for the production of sex hormones and eggs. Zinc is needed to absorb folate. Oysters have the highest concentrations of zinc—one oyster easily supplies a day's worth of zinc. The next highest sources are crustaceans (including shell fish), liver, beef, and pumpkin seeds.

- **Iron** is needed by the egg to make protein and DNA. Iron is found in red meat and the organs of all animals. Vegetable sources like spinach and chocolate are better absorbed in the presence of heme iron (iron from animal sources).

- **Vitamin C** improves fertility in women with luteal phase defect and prevents preterm birth. It is also required for iron absorption.

- **Iodine** is important to prevent miscarriage, unexplained infertility, and many other conditions, including hypothyroidism. Iodine is found in fish, fish roe, and kelp. We only need iodine in small amounts, but the repercussions of deficiency are severe. Since iodine is primarily found in seafood, it has proven a challenge for some people around the world to obtain it. Traditional peoples would go to great lengths to obtain it if no seafood was available. In Africa, some tribes would cook with the ashes of certain plants for their iodine source.

◆ **Bee Propolis**, a substance made by bees, may improve fertility in women with endometriosis.

This is a long list, but don't be overwhelmed. It's really not so complicated. A woman only needs to focus on eating a few primary foods and avoiding a few others to prepare herself for conception.

Foods to Eat Each Day	Foods to Eat Each Week
Fish or meat	Organs from fish or meat
Green leafy vegetables	Shellfish
Avocados	Fish eggs
Citrus	Sea vegetables (can be eaten daily)
Pastured butter, lard, coconut oil	Eggs (can be eaten daily)

Insulin Resistance

Insulin resistance plays another key role in fertility. Too much insulin disrupts the natural balance of hormones. One of the main causes of my own infertility was the inability of my ovaries to mature and release eggs. This is caused when high insulin affects the production of androgens. When androgens are too high and progesterone too low, the egg cannot escape the follicle and will not travel down the fallopian tube. Without an egg coming down the fallopian tube, there can be no fertilization. This and other causes of infertility can be avoided and reversed by avoiding grains, refined carbohydrates, vegetable oils, and by eating a nutrient-dense diet of traditional foods.

Fetal Nutrition

It is a shame I didn't know about traditional foods before I got pregnant with my first child, Evelyn. Ideally, a woman will focus on building up reserves of minerals and fat-soluble vitamins four months to a year before conception even takes place.

Certain nutrients are important for the continuation of the pregnancy and the proper development of the fetus. The job of making a baby from scratch requires a significant amount of nutrients. When a woman is pregnant, she is not simply carrying a baby, she is *manufacturing* one. The mother is not just a warehouse where goods are stored, she is a factory where raw materials must come in so that a product can be produced. On days when a pregnant mother doesn't eat enough of the right foods she will resort to using her own stores. This is no big deal if it only happens occasionally and if the mother has plenty of nutrients to spare. It is a really big deal, however, if the nutrient stores are low to begin with. If there simply is no extra Vitamin A, for example, the baby's eyes will not develop properly. If there are insufficient bone building minerals, the baby's skeleton will suffer. The nutritional deficiencies of the mother predict how healthy the baby will be.

How the Body Borrows Nutrients: The Placenta

The placenta is like a nanny to the baby. When the first mother fails—that's me and you—the second mother comes to the rescue, scavenging for the baby's needs. It's a darn good thing the baby has this nanny, too, because the mother often doesn't know what she should be eating and is sometimes unable to eat what she knows she should. If she is sick and not eating much, if she is busy and not eating properly, the nanny comes to the rescue. The nanny has been entrusted with the job of caring for the baby under any circumstances. If this is at the expense of the mother, so be it—up to a certain point, of course. The job of the placenta is to build the healthiest baby possible without actually killing off the mother. If the mother dies, the mission has totally failed. Without the host there can be no baby. So the placenta is careful about how much nutrients it will extract from the mother.

Pregnancy Demands on the Mother

Eating a nutrient-dense diet before conception not only benefits the baby by giving her the most optimum building blocks for life, it also prepares and protects the mother. After nine months of handing out personal stores of nutrients, the mother's bones can become so soft that her posture is now hunched. Her brain can be literally drained of omega-3 fatty acids, setting her up for depression and cognitive decline. Her skin can look aged, her hair lackluster.

The nutrient requirements it takes to produce a baby can drain the mother of stores of the fat-soluble nutrients like Vitamins A and D, essential fatty acids like DHA, minerals like iron, calcium, potassium, zinc, and magnesium, as well as folate, B12, and selenium. This is why it is so essential for mothers to be vigilant when it comes to nutrition, to be sure that she is replacing what the baby needs.

Child Spacing

No matter how healthy the diet, a mother *will* be depleted in at least some nutrients after the birth of her baby. If she wants to be ready for the next child, she needs time to refuel, both for her own health and for the optimum growth of the baby. While this practice has declined in the modern world, child spacing was the norm among so-called primitive people. The optimum amount of time between children is three years, and the ill effects of conceiving before then is apparent in the bone structure of subsequent children. Catherine Shanahan, MD writes extensively of this phenomenon, called second sibling syndrome, in her wonderful book, *Deep Nutrition: Why Your Genes Need Traditional Food*. Her research, which includes comparing the faces of first children and their siblings, provides compelling evidence of the connection between nutrient stores, the mother's health status, and the bone development of a fetus and child.

The jaws of second children—and children of nutrient depleted mothers in general—are narrower, which leads to crowding of the teeth. The cheekbones are lower, and may not be visible at all, allowing the skin below the eyes to sag and bag. The eyes are spaced closer together. The brow is less prominent and the nose is shorter and narrower. All of these facial attributes can lead to a less attractive person. And it is not just facial bone structure that is compromised. The overall skeleton can be underdeveloped. The bones might turn out smaller and weaker, the legs can be bowed, and women's hips narrowed. This produces weaker adults and women more prone to childbirth problems.

In addition to the problems listed above, the child's brain can be affected by maternal omega-3 deficiency. Second siblings, spaced close together, can have slightly lower IQs.

A Note on Prenatal Vitamins

Multivitamins are best taken pre-conception to improve fertility and to boost nutrient stores for the big job of making a baby out of your own flesh and blood. However, care should be taken when considering nutritional supplements. While prenatal vitamins do offer nutrients needed for health, they should not be substituted for real, fresh foods. Indeed, supplements can sometimes be harmful.

Folic acid, a synthetic variant of folate, is a vitamin found in nearly all prenatal vitamins. Recently, this synthetic variant has been shown to do more harm than good. While it does help to prevent spina bifida, long-term, excessive intake can cause cancer. Iron can cause constipation, a problem from which many pregnant women already suffer. And many other vitamins in prenatal supplements are synthetic, such as Vitamin A, which has been linked to birth defects. (Natural Vitamin A is safe, however.) Vitamin E supplements, as noted above, only include 16 of about 100 isomers.

Since many nutrients work synergistically, multivitamins are in every way inferior to eating real food when it comes to getting the nutrition you need. But if you are going to take vitamins, be sure to get them from a trusted source since many mainstream brands have been shown to be contaminated with toxic compounds such as lead and copper.

So if at all possible, reserve nutritional supplements for supplementation in an area where there is a lack. If you know you don't eat salads as much as you should, for example, taking B6 and folate might be a good idea. If you don't eat fish very often or get enough sunlight, add cod liver oil to your diet.

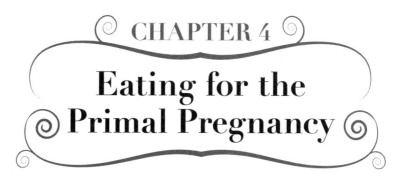

CHAPTER 4

Eating for the Primal Pregnancy

No matter how strong-willed you are, veering away from conventional wisdom when you're pregnant is scary. It's easy to experiment on yourself, but when another little life is involved it becomes serious. You really can't mess this up. I started eating Paleo eight years ago, a few months before Evelyn was conceived, and I was scared, too. I felt like a revolutionary, a daredevil, a weirdo. Now, though, after years of research, I realize that this perception was miles off the mark. It is the Standard America Diet and the FDA-approved food pyramid that is weird, and those following it are the daredevils. The scientists who came up with the food pyramid made a lot of guesses about the very young science of nutrition. They totally ignored tradition and at times even ignored obvious facts. They were led by those funding their "research"—the dairy and agriculture industries.

I am not suggesting that you become a revolutionary, or step out on a limb and attempt something no one has tried before. Quite the opposite. I am asking that you return to the ways of your ancestors and eat the way they ate. By your ancestors, I don't mean your grandparents, whose teeth were likely crooked and full of cavities and whose skin was wrinkled and sagging; I don't mean the original settlers of this country, who undermined the health of the American Indians with small pox and other disease; and I don't mean the Egyptians, whose skeletons were malformed and who suffered many of the diseases we see today. For a peek at vibrant health, we need to look at examples of "uncivilized" groups of people—the hunters and gatherers.

A Safe Return to Ancient Ways

I don't suggest that we return to life as our primitive ancestors knew it—a way of life that did not offer the securities and comforts that we enjoy and depend on today. A complete return to a hunter-gatherer life would mean abandoning everything we've worked thousands of years to achieve. While that is, of course, is not possible, it's also not necessary. We can still achieve vibrant health for ourselves and for our children simply by *emulating* our ancestors. Millions have already proven optimal health is possible right here in the concrete jungle.

I myself was one of the pioneer women of this movement, starting my first Paleo pregnancy before there were any books or websites about it, and before I knew a single soul who followed the same path. But to me, the diet and lifestyle were intuitive and the vibrant health of the hunter-gatherer a real option. Now, after years of following and feeding my family the Primal diet, I am going to teach you what I eat and why. I will also show you how my diet has evolved over the years as I have learned more and more about Paleo nutrition and the diets of traditional women.

For the hunter-gatherer, food was not limited to berries, leaves, and muscle meat. The development of opposable thumbs allowed us to use the tools that enabled us to crack open animal skulls and to extract the rich marrow at the center of bones. Brains and marrow would have been some of the most abundant foods in the ancient world since we were just about the only creature who could get at them. Research suggests that early humans were actually scavengers, not hunters. We would let animal predators do the dirty work, wait for them to clear off, then scavenge for the calorie-rich delicacies they could not extract. The high omega-3 content of marrow and brains contributed to the development of our own brains, which grew larger. And as we got smarter, our ability to procure even more nutritious brain-building foods increased. We learned to harness fire, enabling us to make broth from bones and eat even more meat cooked. We used our dexterity to dig for starch-rich roots, and extract grubs, bugs, and worms. Our increased cunning led to more sophisticated tools and the hunting of larger game. In time, our ancestors became the top species on the planet, able to eat a variety of foods and thrive in virtually any climate.

Nowadays, of course, we are even more adaptable, so the options for a Primal diet are much greater than they were for our ancestors. So how do you begin if you want to go Primal, and, more specifically, if you are pregnant? Let's start with some basic rules. First, stick to the food groups which have been consistently available to humans throughout our history: meat, animal fat, starch, and plants, plus small amounts of nuts, seeds, safe grains, and raw dairy. Second, at all costs, avoid the highly processed foods that are a product of industrialization.

Foods to Always Avoid

- Grain and seed oils like corn and sunflower
- Partially hydrogenated oils
- Pasteurized and homogenized dairy
- Legumes like beans, peanuts, and soy
- Processed meats
- Cereal and oatmeal
- Pasta and bread
- Texturizing gums like xanthan and guar
- Food colorings and flavorings
- Sugar and fruit juice (unless fresh and raw)

Conventional dietary wisdom was developed within the last century by nutritionists who know very little about nutrition—e.g., the low fat movement of the 80s. Traditional wisdom was passed down over thousands of years and is based on instinct and keen observation. Conventional wisdom suggests that eating ample fruits and vegetables is the most important thing a pregnant woman can do. A Google search of "pregnancy nutrition" (which is highly misleading—don't try this at home!) will produce pages of pictures of pregnant women eating fruit, staring at dry salads with a great big smile, and contemplating what to buy in the produce aisle. According to these "experts," being healthy and pregnant is a low-fat, zero-animal fat, nearly vegetarian diet. This conventional American "wisdom" radically contradicts the centuries of actual wisdom acquired by ancient cultures all over the world.

There is much to be learned from the way in which women in traditional cultures prepare for pregnancy. Even before conception, and certainly during the nine months of carrying a child, they eat a highly nutritious diet consisting of special foods that are not always easy to find. (When the special foods are scarce, the tribe's pregnant women always take priority.) These include foods rich in B Vitamins, the fat-soluble Vitamins D, E, and A, plus zinc, and iodine. These vitamins are critical for happy, contented babies with high immunity to disease and should be eaten liberally. Here's where you can find them:

Sources of Fat Soluble Vitamins

- Organs such as liver, heart, and kidney
- Pastured butter and whole fat dairy
- Egg yolks from pastured chickens
- Bone marrow
- Cod liver oil
- Fish eggs
- Avocado
- Olive oil

Meat

Meat offers a lot of value to humans. It is easily digestible and contains some vitamins that cannot be found in vegetables. Although not every hunter-gatherer group ate large amounts of meat, research indicates that they all made an effort to include it in their diet. The type of meat that ancient humans ate, however, was very different from what is commonly available today.

Grass-fed Versus Factory-Farmed Animals

Ancient meat didn't come from animals medicated to control disease. It didn't come from animals that sat in over-crowded, indoor pens fattening up on grain. Farm animals, like cows, are unable to properly digest grain, so their flesh becomes acidic. It is the nutrients from grass that makes their meat nutritious. The meat our ancestors ate came from active animals that lived outside, in open air and sunshine, eating the diet they had evolved to eat. Meat from animals like these nourishes humans. Meat from factory-farmed animals hurts us.

In my experience, much of the published news we see regarding the "dangers" of eating meat are based on poorly executed studies done on subjects eating the worst kind of meat available. I do not recommend eating factory-farmed animals; vibrant health can never be achieved by eating this kind of meat. When I talk of meat, I mean grass-fed, grass-finished animals that have been allowed to graze in a pasture from the time it is weaned until the time it is butchered. Animals that are grass-fed but not grass-finished spend most of their lives that way, but then get switched to grain feedlots before they are butchered.

Organ Meats and Other "Icky" Parts

What parts of an animal should we eat? There is great confusion over this. In the United States, we eat primarily muscle meats; the animal's viscera are generally thrown out. We have all but abandoned the ancient practice of eating organs, also known as "animal by-products." This is unfortunate because the organs, marrow, intestines, and bones are actually the most nutritious parts of the animal. While indulging in a good, rare steak is fine, the multitude of other animal parts should not be left out. The bones are an important source of minerals such as calcium. The liver is replete with iron, Vitamin A, and K2. The connective tissue contains cartilage-forming collagen, which is released in broth.

Some Native Americans threw the muscle meat—the meat we commonly eat—to the dogs, saving the fattier, higher nutrient parts of the animal for themselves. Modern Americans, on the other hand, throw millions of pounds of meat and fish organs away every year. As a result, organs are cheap. If you're trying to figure out how to eat Paleo on a dime, organs are the way to go. They contain all the protein and twice the nutrition of muscle meats.

When we eat animals, we should strive to consume the whole animal: the organs, marrow, eyes, brains, and bones (when used in broth). This may sound odd to Americans, who are accustomed to eating steaks and chicken breast, but it is not strange to the rest of the world. A few years ago, I was in Colombia in South America, were one of the traditions is to suck the eyeballs and brains from fish heads in soup—something I was delighted to participate in. This is not something I've seen in the US; I imagine most people here would find that practice repulsive. But in Colombia, it would be considered weird to throw out the fish heads, just as it would be weird for a hunter-gatherer to throw out a delicacy like offal. Even weirder to them? Zapping a box of frozen "edibles" in the microwave.

How to Properly Cook Meat

Traditional people around the world typically eat some of their animal products raw (including liver, seafood, and milk), but when it comes to muscle meat it has to be softened to be digestible. Marinating, fermenting, and cooking are methods we can use to achieve this. When it comes to cooking, moisture, either from water or fat, yields a healthier product. When we boil meat, the moisture trapped inside slices the strands of protein during the cooking process; this is called hydrolytic cleavage, which we refer to as tenderizing. Additionally, the trapped water prevents proteins from fusing together, which is what makes the meat much less digestible.

Cooking muscle meat at more than 300 degrees and with dry heat toughens the meat and creates carcinogens like heterocyclic amines and polycyclic aromatic hydrocarbons (PAH). The latter are formed when fat and juices drip from a grill or open fire, and the flames that result, which contain PAH, adhere to the surface of the meat.

Meat is a nearly complete source of nutrients for humans when eaten as a whole animal, but care must be taken: Know how your meat was raised and make sure it is cooked properly, whether you or someone else makes it.

Animal Fat

Humans have always consumed the fatty animal parts. We started favoring lean chicken breast and skim milk as a misconceived response to obesity and heart disease, but that was not the way our ancient ancestors ate. Fat is high in calories and, when you're eating to survive, calories are a virtue not a vice. We evolved into the creatures we are today because we ate animal fat and, as a result, our bodies have come to depend on it. Fat is required to produce sex hormones and to absorb fat-soluble vitamins. Fat also comprises the bulk of the cell membrane for every cell in our body. We cannot function without fats in our diets, but it has to be the *right* kinds of fat.

While low fat diets are still popular among weight loss enthusiasts, the trend has moved from low fat to "healthy fats." According to the American Heart Association, saturated and trans fats cause heart disease and raise cholesterol as well as make you fat; monounsaturated and polyunsaturated fats, on the other hand, they say are "better alternatives" and help lower cholesterol and prevent heart disease.

This recommendation is flat out wrong. It's also the same recommendation given by nearly all doctors and scientists in the United States, and it has landed us in a world of trouble. While it is true that fats contain more calories per gram than carbohydrates or protein, it is not true that fat makes you fat. In fact, fat—and especially cholesterol—is highly satiating and helps to curb cravings and control appetite, unlike carbohydrates. The "better" vegetable oils, which the American Medical Association (AMA) claims lower cholesterol and prevent heart disease, do just the opposite.

Cholesterol

High serum cholesterol can act as a *marker* for heart disease in predisposed individuals, but it is not the cause. This is where scientists went wrong. They assumed that cholesterol was a causative factor in heart disease when, in reality, it is sometimes simply *associated* with heart disease.

The Real Cause of High Cholesterol

Serum cholesterol rises when cells become damaged, not the other way around. High cholesterol does not itself cause cellular damage. Scar tissue, for example, contains a lot of cholesterol, but the cholesterol wasn't the cause of the wound; it was sent to help repair the wound. Likewise, damaged arteries attract cholesterol to help them heal. So taking drugs to lower cholesterol is like sending the medics home during a war—not a genius strategy.

Cellular wounds can take place in a number of ways. Free radicals, viruses, and damaged dietary cholesterol can all cause wounds on a cellular level. Free radicals and viruses damage cells on a regular basis. In response, the body sends cholesterol to the site to heal it. This is the body's natural process and it works very well in healthy people, but when the cholesterol that is sent in is damaged cholesterol, the cells are in for a world of hurt. The damaged cholesterol does even more harm to the already injured cells.

Sources of Damaged Dietary Cholesterol

- Powdered milk
- Skim milk (powdered milk is added for body)
- Powdered eggs
- Whipped cream
- Ultra-pasteurized cream and milk
- Homogenized milk
- Overcooked meats
- Rancid and burned fats

Cholesterol is a reparative substance that the body especially needs in the presence of stress or a bad diet. In fact, it has myriad benefits beyond repairing damaged tissues:

1. Cholesterol makes cells thicker and improves the stability of the cell membrane.

2. Cholesterol is a precursor to Vitamin D. Sunshine reacts with the cholesterol in our skin to produce the bone-building vitamin, Vitamin D.

3. Cholesterol is a precursor to corticosteroids and sex hormones. Without cholesterol, our stress response may be poor and our sex hormone production low.

4. Cholesterol protects against infections.

5. Cholesterol helps you to feel full.

6. Bile salts, which help assimilate fats, are made from cholesterol. Without bile salts, we don't digest fat properly and, hence, don't absorb fat-soluble nutrients.

7. Cholesterol makes you happier. Jay Kaplan, PhD, director of the Wake Forest University Primate Center, showed that monkeys with lower cholesterol are more aggressive. The lack of cholesterol in the brain's cell membranes affects the function of serotonin receptors. Serotonin is one of the brain's happy chemicals.

Vegetable Oils

With the exception of coconut oil, which can easily be extracted from coconut meat by fermentation, and olive oil, which can be cold-pressed from olives, vegetable oils are difficult to make—way too difficult for hunter-gatherers. But even the relatively easier and nutrient-preserving processes for extracting olive and coconut oils are relatively new to human history (one theory dates olive oil extraction to 4500 BC). Still, we generally consider these oils to be good for us since the saturated fats in coconut oil and the monounsaturated fats in olive oil are present and abundant in nature, and our bodies have evolved to utilize them with no trouble. But other "vegetable oils" (which are grain, legume, and seed oils) don't have the fatty acid composition that is right for our bodies and therefore don't confer the same benefits. In fact, they do us quite a bit of harm, as we shall see.

Harmful "Vegetable Oils"	
Corn (grain)	Cottonseed (seed)
Soybean (legume)	Sunflower (seed)
Peanut (legume)	Safflower (seed)
Sesame (seed)	Canola (seed)

To produce these seed, legume and grain oils—which really shouldn't be called vegetable oils at all—they must be heated or chemically processed using the poisonous solvent hexane, and then must undergo additional processes to remove hexane's foul stench. Hexane processing strips all of the nutrients from the extracted oil and oxidizes the delicate polyunsaturated fatty acids (PUFAs), rendering them poisonous to our bodies. Oils like these would never have been used by our ancestors. They are not something they could have even produced and, hence, they are not something we evolved to utilize.

Undamaged PUFAs are not widely available in nature and oxidized PUFAs even less so. As a result, our bodies are not adapted to process them in large quantities. When we eat a diet high in PUFAs, they wind up taking the place of other fats in our cells. And instead of strengthening us, these seed oils weaken our bodies' systems.

For example, when our diet contains a high amount of seed and grain oils, the polyunsaturated fatty acids begin to replace the saturated fatty acids in our cell membranes. Saturated fatty acids are what make our cells strong and stiff. They comprise at least 50 percent of our cell membranes. PUFAs are flexible, due to their missing carbon atoms on the fatty acid chain. When they replace saturated fatty acids in our cells, our cells become weak. What happens when cells are weak? Cholesterol to the rescue! Cholesterol must come in to work on the damage. This temporarily lowers serum cholesterol as the cholesterol is now mobilized to do a job. This is one reason why vegetable oils appear to lower serum cholesterol. But as we can see, this temporary reduction is not actually a sign of good health; rather, it is a sign of a body in distress. And when that mobilized cholesterol is oxidized cholesterol, the situation gets even worse—our cells endure even greater damage.

We should avoid all seed oils for two reasons: they have high omega-6 content and the processing has oxidized them. Other than moderate doses of the healing cold-pressed oils like coconut and olive (and perhaps flax), vegetable oils cause harm. Animal fat, on the other hand, helps our skin remain youthful, our hormones to be naturally balanced, and our moods to be even. Animal fat should not be avoided—not in pregnancy or ever.

Some Telling Statistics

Animal fat has been so successfully vilified here in the US that we now consider it an indulgence. In reality, of course, the truth is quite the contrary. It is the polyunsaturated fats (from grain and seed oils) that are indulgent and destructive. Saturated and monounsaturated fats are the most abundant and accessible in the natural world and they are the fats we evolved to need. Without saturated and monounsaturated fats we either couldn't eat fat at all or would have to rely on the assistance of modern "food" processing, as many of us do. But this is not something that was even possible 100 years ago. Our ancestors didn't eat a fat-free diet, they ate the fats that were available to them—animal fats.

I see the move towards "vegetable" oils and away from animal fats as nothing short of brainwashing, brought on primarily by profit-driven corporations. Granted, bad science and hearsay also helped spread the myth, but the corporations selling these products have it in their interest to keep the myth alive. This effort is proving to have devastating long-term consequences. Because of the industrialization of our food supply and our move away from farms and into cities, the majority of Americans now suffer from heart disease, cancer, arthritis, and other formerly rare conditions.

According to the CDC (Center for Disease Control), heart disease accounted for approximately 7 percent of all deaths in 1900. By 1930, the percentage had risen to 18 percent. And then it really started climbing: By 1940, it was up to 27 percent, and by the next decade it was hovering around 35 percent, where it remained through the 1990s.

This data is telling when you consider the history of vegetable oils. In 1911, Proctor and Gamble began selling Crisco, the hydrogenated shortening produced from cottonseeds. This was an inventively cheap alternative to butter and it made a fortune for the company, until the recent exposure of the health hazards of trans fats. In the 1930s, soybean oil started to become popular and there was a big jump in the number of heart related deaths as soon as 1940; by 1950, soybean oil had become the most popular cooking oil. Even today, vegetable oils of various types (canola is the most hyped now) have almost totally replaced animal fats, and heart disease-related deaths remain high.

Starch and Fruit

Starch

There is much debate in the Primal/Paleo communities about the inclusion of starches in an ancestral diet. It's a debate that won't end soon. Those opposed to starch argue that ancient man ate a low carbohydrate diet and would have been in ketosis most of the time, i.e. he would have utilized fat for energy with more efficiency than most of us today do. Others contend that foraging for starch would not have been as difficult as hunting and would have been the most calorie rich food available when meat was scarce, making it a food that we likely evolved to eat. Archaeological evidence is limited and so the debate goes on.

If indeed ancient man did eat starch, which I believe to be true since we see so much evidence of it in modern hunter-gatherers, how do we eat similarly? Unlike them, we aren't pulling down starchy trees, scraping out the middle, and fermenting the contents. We aren't foraging wild tubers. So what do we eat then when our choices are limited to modern agriculture? If we can't realistically seek out the exact same foods as hunter-gatherers, we can opt for alternatives that do no harm. These alternatives have recently been dubbed "safe starches." Here are some that are easily acquired:

Safe Starches for the Primal Diet:

- **Sweet potatoes** and yams are virtually free of anti-nutrients and are high in beta-carotene and other nutrients.

- **Plantain**, a relative of the banana, is like a starchy vegetable and only develops sweetness when very ripe.

- **Yuca**, a tropical starch, is native to South America and known as cassava in other tropical regions.

- **Tapioca** is the extracted starch of yucca or cassava.

- **Sago** is a starch extracted from palm trees in New Guinea and the East Indies. It is used in cooking and made into pearls for pudding.

- **Taro** is a starchy root vegetable used around the world and a traditional staple of Hawaii.

- **Chestnuts**, unripened, are a starchy tree fruit common around Christmas time.

- **White potatoes** may not be considered safe (depending on who you ask) because they are nightshades and contain the poison glycoalkaloid. Note, however, that this chemical is in much higher concentrations when the root is green.

- **White rice**, though it is a grain, is considered a safe starch.

Some of these starches are refined, like white rice, sago, and tapioca. While they do have a high glycemic index, extracted starches are common among some hunter-gatherers. This may be problematic for anyone who is metabolically challenged due to an industrialized diet, however. If so, avoid the spikes in blood sugar and delay gastric emptying by combining these foods with meat, fish, fats, or vegetables, rather than eating them on their own.

Starches considered unsafe are corn, quinoa, brown rice, oats, and others which contain phytic acid; wheat, which contains phytic acid and gluten (and is in many other ways unacceptable in its modern form). The late

Weston A. Price, who wrote the 1939 book *Nutrition and Physical Degeneration* and spent decades traveling through primitive lands, observed that these toxins could be broken down with fermentation and germination—processes that are absolutely necessary to avoid nutrient deficiencies. For many of us, though, even this extra processing does not yield a healthful food.

For healthy people, phytic acid ingested in small doses has not been shown to cause any serious problems. But in the modern diet, phytic acid is taken in rather high doses, especially after whole grains became popular. Whole grains (e.g., wheat, oat, barley, spelt, kamut, rye, and millet) are loaded with anti-nutrients and should be avoided.

For a healthy person there is nothing wrong with including carbohydrates in the diet, and for pregnant women it is advisable. But carbs can quickly cause hormonal imbalances if you eat too much (the carbo-loading in modern diets was impossible for primitive people and, hence our bodies did not evolve to tolerate it). It's hard to say exactly how much carbohydrate our ancient ancestors ate, and it likely varied by region, season, and time in history, but we can determine our ideal range based on science and our own energy levels. 50 to 100 grams of carbohydrates per day is generally recommended for a non-pregnant woman eating a Primal-type diet. This amount provides the brain with necessary glucose and the muscles with glycogen, without leading to metabolic dysfunction. Where you actually fall within this range depends on your activity levels, your stress levels (both physical and emotional), and how much protein you eat.

Pregnant and breastfeeding women have slightly higher glucose requirements. In addition to their own needs, they must feed the baby's brain with a steady stream of glucose or fill the breast milk with lactose. How many carbohydrates a pregnant or breastfeeding woman needs will also depend on her activity and stress levels. If you currently eat 22% of you calories as carbohydrates—for example, 100 grams of a 1800 calorie diet—then increase your carbs proportionately as you increase your calorie needs for pregnancy. So, if your caloric needs increase by 300 calories while you are pregnant, then add 22% of 300 as carbs, so about 16 grams, or one serving.

In the Paleo community, fear of grains and carbohydrates often leads to a total abandonment of starches. This happens for two reasons. The first is that many of us choose to go Primal to lose weight or because of metabolic health related problems and, in that regard, lowering carbohydrate intake is helpful. The second is based on the misconception that ancient humans had no regular access to starches. I do not agree with this theory. Recognizing and acquiring starches is easy. In the north, they can even be stored through the cold season.

As a result of eschewing starches, Paleo diet adherents tend to add a lot of fruit. This, unfortunately, is the route I took while I was pregnant with Evelyn. Fruit is packed with nutrients and antioxidants, but excessive consumption can be harmful.

Fruit

Fruit, like starch, offers ample calories and it packs a nutritional punch, but there are problems with high consumption. Fruit contains a lot of sugar, and excesses of fruit sugar cause hyperactivity and weak tooth enamel. It also has long-term consequences on the liver. Current hunter-gatherers are aware of these side effects; even those who live in tropical regions where fruit is plentiful eat it in moderate quantities and as part of a diet that includes starch, fish, and meat. I would advise limiting fruit to one or two servings per day, and stick, if possible, to varieties that are in season.

Vegetables

Most Paleo writers (and health writers in general) advocate the consumption of large amounts of vegetables. I don't think this is sound advice. First, while plants can offer some of the same nutrients as high-caloric organ meats, they don't provide enough calories, particularly for pregnant women. Second, the nutrients of many plants are bound to indigestible fiber and toxins.

Plant Toxins

While plants are susceptible to getting trampled and yanked out of the ground, they are not totally helpless. They come equipped with their own potent defense system—something even more effective than spines, thorns, or hard shells: poisons. Yes, even many edible plants contain poisons. The nightshades (potatoes, tomatoes, chili peppers), for example, contain natural insecticides, which are poisonous even to us. Other plants contain carcinogens, enzyme inhibitors, neurotoxins, and allergens. Plants can be dangerous unless you are a species with a built-in ability to neutralize these poisons, or one with a big enough brain to sidestep their defenses with simple technology. Like us. Throughout human history, we have been deactivating poisonous plant compounds through the processes of cooking, fermentation, and sprouting. Some vegetables are okay to eat raw while others are better after some form of processing. However, even then, vegetables are high in fiber, which can be damaging in high doses.

Fiber

Plant matter is indigestible by our bodies, and too much of it interferes with the absorption of nutrients. This problem can be circumvented, however, through fermentation, a process that breaks down the fibers and releases trapped nutrients. Some research indicates that fiber in excess of 30 grams per day impairs the absorption of nutrients. For anyone with a weakened digestive tract, even that much can be irritating.

If your digestive system is damaged or if you don't like vegetables, organ meats, bone broths, and seafood offer similar, if not superior, nutrition without the plant toxins and high fiber. However, many nutrients are quite abundant in vegetables, like magnesium, potassium, B Vitamins, soluble fiber, and Vitamin C. As long as they are not eaten in excess, vegetables are a tasty way to supplement the diet and ensure optimal nutrition for you and your baby.

Nuts and Seeds

Nuts and seeds are coated with phytic acid—a useful protection for them, but damaging for us. Raw nuts and seeds *can* be eaten fresh from the shell in very small amounts or as more substantial snacks if they are first either germinated or soaked in water cultured with lactic acid. Although nuts are tasty when roasted, opt for raw (and preferably still in the shell) because high heats ruin the polyunsaturated fats of most nuts.

The Problem with Phytates and Phytic Acid

Phytic acid is a type of storage molecule for phosphorous, whose chemical structure is such that it also binds to calcium, zinc, iron, and magnesium. In this form, the compound is called a phytate. Many plants contain these mineral-binding compounds. They are present in grains, nuts, seeds, and legumes, and some have a higher content than others.

Phytates play an important role in the life of a seed. They hold the necessary phosphorus in stasis until the seed is ready for germination. This is why seeds can sit for ages without becoming a plant. Everything they need is bound up as phytates until the time is right for germination. This is great for the seed but not so good for us when we eat it in its whole, raw form. The presence of large amounts of phytic acid in our diets can cause significant harm by making minerals unavailable for absorption and inhibiting digestive enzymes. That in turn makes it difficult to digest protein and carbohydrates. As a result, eating too much phytic acid can cause tooth decay, osteoporosis, and rickets.

Foods with High Levels of Phytates:

- Unfermented soy products like tofu and soymilk
- Raw cocoa and cheap coffee
- Nuts
- Seeds
- Peanuts
- Whole grain bread, especially unleavened
- Corn and corn products like tortillas
- Oats and oatmeal
- Beans
- Chickpeas

Many people, such as vegetarians and those who cannot afford to eat much meat, depend on these foods for the protein they contain. People adopting alternative raw food diets are encouraged to eat these foods in their whole, unadulterated state. And people turning to Paleo to improve their health load up with nut and seed butters, as well as a variety of alternative nut-based baked goods to add variety to their diets. As a result, they are consuming a lot of phytic acid and doing their bodies harm. It would take traditional food preparation practices (which I detail below) to make these foods healthy. Preparing these foods in the home is the only way to ensure their safety. Food manufacturers would rather cut cost and produce products faster, than follow procedures for reducing the harmful compounds.

At first glance, nut-based baked goodies seems like a smart way to cheat the system—as long as the ingredients are Paleo, you can have your cake and eat it too, right? But these "Paleo products" are only Paleo if they are eaten occasionally and in small amounts. While making a switch to ancestral eating can be difficult at first, these treats can be dangerous, causing everything from tooth decay and stunted growth due to the lack of bone-building nutrients, to digestive distress caused by the inactivity of digestive enzymes. If you are trying to recover from any kind of digestive dysfunction, which most of us are these days, nut flour products will only set you back. And if you are hoping to maintain a healthy diet and lifestyle, over-consumption of nuts can damage a once healthy digestive tract and deplete nutrient stores.

Getting the Phytic Acid Out of the Food

There are a few ways to release phytates from their duty to bind nutrients:

- Phytase enzymes released during germination
- Stomach acid, to some degree
- The phytase enzyme activity in lactobacillus
- Roasting (can reduce phytic acid by 40%)

Soaking induces sprouting which can release, reduce, or even totally eliminate the phytic acid content in many—but not all—raw seeds, nuts, grains, and legumes. For example, brown rice, millet, corn, and oats do not contain sufficient phytase for soaking of the grain to do any good. These foods must be soaked in an acid medium—lemon juice, vinegar, or whey—to eliminate the phytic acid. Nuts and seeds contain varying levels of phytic acid—some of them quite high—and so do coffee, cocoa powder, and most commercially prepared soy sauces. Cheap coffee, non-traditionally prepared soy sauce, and raw cocoa powder are particularly harmful because they have not undergone the necessary fermentation process to remove phytic acid. Using these regularly can have detrimental effects on mineral absorption.

Sally Fallon, a traditional foods advocate and author of *Nourishing Traditions*, has done her own research on the best and most effective way to soak nuts. She suggests soaking nuts in salt water and then drying them at a low temperature, following the ways of traditional South American natives. Research is inconclusive as to how effective the process is but observation suggests that nuts become much more digestible when soaked in salt water overnight and then dried out on a baking sheet in an oven no hotter than 150 degrees. The nuts should be turned occasionally and should be let to dry thoroughly so that they don't go bad during storage.

Pregnant women should be particularly concerned about phytic acid because of the body's increased demand for nutrients. In a study published in the *American Journal of Clinical Nutrition*, researchers at the University of the Witwatersrand, Johannesburg, South Africa compared iron absorption of Indian women who ate nut meal breads with Indian women who ate white grain breads. The team found that iron absorption was significantly reduced in the group eating nut bread. They noted that the two main promoters of iron absorption were ascorbic acid (Vitamin C) and meat.

Fermentation

The specific anti-nutrient content in foods really isn't important. All we need to know is how to tame the anti-nutritional beast. And that is quite simple; people have been doing it for thousands of years. The process is fermentation: the breakdown of molecules, via friendly bacteria and yeasts, which renders foods more nutritious and easier to digest.

History of Fermented Foods

Since nobody had refrigeration before the twentieth century, and fermentation is inevitable without it, every traditional culture around the world has its own signature fermented food. For Russians, it's *kefir*, a thick, yeast-fermented milk. For the Chinese it's the *thousand-year egg*, a nearly black, preserved egg. For Koreans, it's *kimchi*, a pungent side dish of fermented cabbage, garlic, and peppers. Colombians drink a fermented corn beverage called *chicha*. Germans eat sauerkraut, or fermented cabbage. A staple food for Hawaiians is *poi*, a fermented taro porridge. The Japanese add the sticky and stinky fermented soybeans called *natto* on top of rice. And *kombucha*, a fermented tea, has been adopted by cultures all over the world.

The fermentation of foods is both the natural course of food as it spoils, and a deliberate method of preservation. If you leave raw milk out, for example, the naturally present lactobacillus turns it into yogurt. When you soak nuts in warm water, yeasts are mobilized to start the process of breaking them down. Making mead, a honey wine, is as simple as adding water to honey and letting the natural yeasts present in the honey do their magic. The same is true of grape wine. The yeasts present on the skin of the grape transform the sweet fruit into wine.

Benefits of Fermented Foods

Fermented foods should *always* be a part of a healthy diet. Friendly bacteria and yeasts confer so many benefits, we simply cannot be healthy without them. We are designed to work in synergy with microbes. Scientists discover new benefits all the time. Some of these include:

- Fermentation neutralizes plant toxins.
- Fermentation of foods releases trapped vitamins and minerals from plant fibers.
- Bacteria and yeasts are replete with B Vitamins.
- Bacteria help to stimulate peristalsis (fecal elimination).

- Friendly bacteria keep pathogens from gaining territory in our gut, keeping us from getting sick.

- Friendly bacteria, which travels through the vaginal canal during birth, increases the serotonin levels in the brain in adulthood. Serotonin is a neurotransmitter responsible for making us feel happy. This relationship highlights the importance of vaginal births over cesarean, in addition to the importance of the mother maintaining healthy vaginal flora while pregnant.

One of the biggest health problems of a Western diet is the exclusion of fermented foods in favor of foods that are dead. Juices and bagged, boxed, canned, and irradiated foods are all designed to be sterile so that pathogens don't grow during storage. While this keeps us from getting food poisoning in the short run, it makes us more susceptible to sickness in the long run by weakening our immune systems.

Healthy Flora Can Prevent Neonatal Infections

Fermented foods are important for everyone, and critical for the pregnant woman. When a baby is born vaginally, he or she is inoculated with the mother's flora. The mother can confer a strong immune system to her baby just by having healthy intestinal flora herself. But if the mother's flora is off balance due to an overgrowth of pathogens, the baby can inherit this, too. Many bacterial infections are passed from mother to baby in the birth canal. Some of these infections include: streptococcus B, listeriosis, E. coli, sepsis, meningitis, and candidiasis. Many are serious, requiring hospitalization, while others cause less noticeable problems, such as poor feeding, listlessness, skin rashes, irritability, and persistent crying. These can generally be avoided by improving the mother's gut ecology during pregnancy.

Dairy

Many people think of dairy as a product of agriculture—probably because dairy animals as we know them live in pens and eat the grain provided in troughs. In reality, agriculture should have nothing at all to do with dairy animals, as ruminants (mammals that digest by chewing and rechewing food, breaking it down bacterially—like cows, sheep, goats, and deer) are relatively easy to herd and are not designed to eat anything but plant-based foods.

The Diet of a Ruminant

Cows were designed to pull nutrition from grasses and other low-lying leafy greens. The process is very specialized and requires the use of four stomachs for the breakdown of the plants and the assimilation of their nutrients. In a ruminant's stomach, grass undergoes a whole lot of fermentation to get at the sugars and proteins used for energy. This specialized digestive system isn't designed to break down meat or starch or seeds or nuts. When a cow is given these other foods, like grains, problems arise. Grains contain starch. Since cows were designed to ferment grasses, starch undergoes wild fermentation on the long journey through the gut, ultimately becoming acidic. This acidity contributes to making the animal sick and susceptible to disease.

Cows who graze in pastures present a very different picture. They are rarely sick and do not require regular doses of antibiotics to survive. The average life of a cow from Organic Pastures, a raw dairy farm in California, is 10 to 12 years, whereas a conventional dairy cow averages 3.5 years. Cows on pasture have robust immune systems as a result of their natural diet and lifestyle.

Effects on the Dairy

The superior quality of the milk is proof of the benefits of pastured living conditions. The high Vitamin A content of pastured butter is apparent in the bright yellow color of the butter. The low Vitamin A content of conventional butter is obvious by the lack of color (unless color is added). The same is true for cheeses. Cheddar cheese from conventional cattle must have annatto added to give it the familiar orange look; cheddar made from grass-fed cows has a naturally appetizing yellow color.

The dairy produced by these nutrient deficient cattle is lower in—even totally devoid of—many of the nutrients that used to be present in our dairy foods. Today, conventional dairy products are devoid of CLA (conjugated linoleic acid) and omega-3s, and are significantly lower in anti-oxidant vitamins such as Vitamin E, A, and selenium.

Ancient Pastoral Societies

Dairy is not, strictly speaking, a Paleolithic food, but it most likely has a longer history in the human diet than grains. Humans may have begun herding dairy animals as early as 30,000 years ago. In Africa, Mongolia, and Norway, there are still semi-nomadic people who live and travel with their animals, and evidence suggests they have done this for tens of thousands of years. The milk is usually fermented or turned into a cheese because it cannot be refrigerated. As milk warms, it sours quickly, which is what fermenting is. The souring process breaks down the proteins and sugars, making them more nutritious and the nutrients more bioavailable. There is ample evidence that dairy foods are remarkably beneficial to health, especially during pregnancy and in early childhood. I defend its use because the traditional peoples who have used and continue to use dairy as a staple have been remarkably robust, exhibiting excellent bone structure, superb dental health, and freedom from most modern disease.

Dairy as we know it in America, however, is not something I would recommend consuming. Unless you can get dairy from a small farm that is very careful to emulate old practices, it will probably do more harm than good. Dairy cows and goats must be fed fresh grass and only hay when supplementation is necessary. They should not be fed grains. The milk should not be homogenized—a process which speeds and breaks down fat molecules through a very fine screen so that the molecules become evenly distributed throughout the milk rather than rising to the top. This process potentially renders the fats toxic to the body. This kind of milk—nearly all milk sold in US stores today—should be avoided. The best milk products come from grass-fed cows and are not homogenized or pasteurized.

Getting Adequate Calcium without Dairy

While dairy is life giving to many, it isn't for everyone. People who are lactose intolerant are not able to break down milk sugar. This causes a disruption in intestinal flora. Some people have allergies to casein, a milk protein. This allergy is common in those who drink high-heat pasteurized and homogenized milk. Still others don't believe in the philosophy of drinking the milk of another mammal.

Avoiding dairy during my first pregnancy was probably the decision that made me most uncomfortable. How could I get enough calcium to feed my growing baby? But then I asked myself, *What did people do for calcium before we started herding animals?* And what about modern hunter-gatherers, who don't herd animals, and other cultures that traditionally don't eat dairy?

After a little thought, it seemed kind of odd that dairy was considered *necessary* during pregnancy. AmericanPregnancy.org recommends 1000 mg of calcium per day for pregnant women, which translates into roughly 3-4 servings of dairy per day. Was this some kind of American nutritional fallacy...

again? Raw dairy might be great for some people, but is it really necessary for all people?

After doing research on the subject, I determined it wasn't. There are millions of healthy people in the world who don't eat dairy. Asians (other than those from India) didn't eat it until recently, and most Asians still don't include it in their diet. The same is true for tribes in the Amazon rain forest. Traditional Hawaiians don't eat dairy either. These are all remarkably healthy people with strong bones and even less incidence of osteoporosis than we have here in the US. So it seems that on the Paleo diet we should be fine without milk, right? Definitely, and as long as we eat other foods that contain calcium. In fact, we might even be better off without it since the calcium-to-magnesium ratio in dairy is very high. Excess calcium can actually cause magnesium loss. That's not necessarily a reason to avoid dairy, but it is a reason to increase your magnesium intake if you do eat dairy.

Doesn't High Protein Intake Cause Calcium Loss?

Maybe you've heard that calcium intake needs to be higher in people who eat more protein, like those of us eating a Primal diet. Well, if you have, there's no need to worry. Upon closer inspection by scientists, this doesn't seem to be the case.

Bones aren't the compact calcium sticks many believe them to be. In fact, bones are composed of 50 percent protein and 50 percent minerals. So, we need substantial amounts of both to make and heal bones. In a 2002 study called *Protein and Calcium: Antagonists or Synergists*, Robert P. Heaney of Creighton University studied the effects of protein and calcium on bone density. He found that subjects who ate less protein suffered more bone loss. According to Heaney, "Those with the highest protein intakes gained bone, whereas those with the lowest intakes actually lost bone. Clearly, calcium was not enough to protect the skeleton when protein intakes were low. Equally clearly, high protein intake did not adversely affect bone status."

He did find that urinary calcium was higher in subjects with a higher protein intake, but that doesn't cause bone loss. When urinary calcium excretion hits 30 mg., our parathyroid gland responds with the excretion of parathyroid hormone, which in turn improves calcium absorption efficiency.

Raw Milk Has Served Primitive Peoples Well

Raw milk from cows grazing on green pasture has served traditional people very well for centuries, if not millennia. The Masai tribe in Africa is an example of a robust and exceptionally tall people who live almost exclusively on raw milk (mostly fermented), meat, and blood. Weston A. Price studied healthy milk-drinking people all over the world and found strong teeth and excellent bone structure among them.

Nevertheless, dairy isn't required for good health. Plenty of women continue to build babies without it. I did. I'm doing it again now. So, how do we get the calcium we need? By turning to other calcium-rich foods, in addition to foods that aid in the absorption of calcium. Bone broth is full of minerals, including calcium. Eggshells are high in calcium and can be dried and then pulverized and added to food. Vitamin D and magnesium both aid in the absorption of calcium.

High Calcium, Dairy-Free Foods

- Spinach, cooked—½ cup, 125 mg
- Bok Choy—½ cup, 80 mg
- Kale, cooked—½ cup, 80 mg
- Collard greens—½ cup, 175 mg
- Molasses—1 tbsp., 40 mg
- Orange—1 large Florida, 64 mg
- Canned salmon with bones—3 oz., 180 mg
- Oysters—3 oz., 80 mg
- Eggs—2 eggs, 50 mg
- Almonds—1 oz., 75 mg
- Brazil nuts—1 oz., 45 mg
- Macadamia nuts—1oz., 23 mg

Sample Calcium-Rich Menu

- **Breakfast**: An orange with two eggs—114 mg
- **Snack**: Some almonds with molasses—135 mg
- **Lunch**: One can of salmon with spinach salad—400 mg
- **Dinner**: Bone broth soup with collard greens—175mg (plus the calcium content of bone broth)
- **Total**: 824 mg (plus the calcium content of bone broth)

What About Sushi?

In the United States, raw fish is considered off limits for pregnant women. But in Japan, raw fish is part of good neonatal nutrition. The Japanese are fanatical about health and cleanliness. Yet pregnant Japanese women have been eating raw fish for centuries, and history has served them well. Why should they change now? In America, the taboo against eating raw fish while pregnant is largely due to our overactive imaginations and fear of foodborne illness.

In my opinion, these fears are unfounded. For one thing, parasites are not present in most types of sushi. They are most common in mollusks like oysters and clams. The National Academy of Sciences Institute of Medicine concluded in a 1991 report about seafood-caused illness that, "most seafood-associated illness is reported from consumers of raw bivalve mollusks. ...The majority of incidents are due to consumption of shellfish from fecally polluted water."

As we know, we should be careful about the origin of our raw seafood. We should never consume raw seafood from polluted waters or seafood farms. That said, the fish generally used in sushi is not the type of fish that harbors parasites. Tuna, for example, is not susceptible because it lives in very cold, deep water. Sushi restaurants generally use farmed salmon because, unlike its wild counterpart, it does not carry parasites. In addition, sushi-grade fish is frozen before it is prepared, and parasites are destroyed with freezing. Is the fact that it's served raw and uncooked dangerous? As the Institute of Medicine reports, food poisoning usually occurs when food is cooked and then cross-contaminated either by dirty hands or through contact with raw product. Cooked food is also at risk of growing pathogens when it isn't served immediately, like when it sits waiting to be picked up by a busy server at a restaurant. In sushi restaurants, where the sushi bar is kept at the proper cold temperature and meticulously cleaned, this factor is not a problem.

Sushi is not only safe for pregnant women, it's healthy. Cooking destroys some amount of nutrients and all of the enzymes. If the fish is cooked "well done," the cooking process denatures the protein, destroys delicate polyunsaturated fats, and creates carcinogens.

What About Alcohol?

Conventional wisdom and the Surgeon General say that drinking alcohol while pregnant causes birth defects. It does if alcohol is drunk often and in large quantities. There is, however, no evidence that drinking the occasional small glass of wine in the second and third trimester causes any ill effects. That doesn't mean that drinking alcohol is perfectly safe, but plenty of healthy pregnant women have enjoyed the occasional glass of wine without harming the baby.

But Is It Primal?

Alcohol, as we know it, is a product of agriculture. And while it's true that any food containing sugar can ferment, the alcohol that results from just letting some fruit rot (which is the only way cavemen could make alcohol) is usually pretty scant. So it's unlikely that Paleolithic men and women were getting drunk on a regular basis. (All you have to do is look at the effects of fetal alcohol syndrome—smaller heads, facial abnormalities, and impaired motor skills—to know that heavy drinking would have put a stop to human evolution as we know it.) Personally, I have no taste for alcohol when I'm pregnant. But I think the occasional glass of wine is fine, as long as it's after the first trimester, when the baby's brain is better protected.

Eating Organic

Eating organic is an important consideration for a pregnant woman. Organic produce contains much higher levels of nutrients than conventionally grown produce, and is free of the harmful chemicals present in produce treated with pesticides.

Nutrition

Two pieces of fruit may appear identical and taste very similar, but when one is organic and one conventionally grown they have very different nutritional profiles. One report showed that organic crops have significantly more Vitamin C, iron, magnesium, and phosphorus. When a mother eats organic produce, she gets more nutrition for herself and her growing baby.

Organic produce is nutritionally superior because of the dirt it grows in. Farms that do not use chemicals have a wider diversity of microbes living in the soil. As we just learned, microbes (bacteria, yeast, and fungi) help to break down plant matter and provide nutrients. This same phenomenon happens in the dirt, which gives the roots more nutrients to absorb, and that gives the plant more nutrition to offer us.

Pesticides

The chemicals in pesticides are incredibly toxic, both to the mother and her baby. While eating a nice juicy peach doesn't appear to cause any ill effects—nobody keels over and instantly dies—the body changes slowly in ways which cause damage to the baby's genes and nutritional status (as you will see in the next chapter.) The changes are also detrimental to the mother's hormones, which can affect her ability to carry her baby to term and bounce back from pregnancy.

According to research conducted by the Environmental Working Group, some fruits and vegetables are higher in pesticides than others. If purchasing 100 percent organic produce is too expensive, at least avoid the products on this Dirty Dozen list of the most contaminated conventionally grown fruits and vegetables.

The Dirty Dozen

- Apples
- Celery
- Peaches
- Spinach
- Lettuce
- Potatoes
- Strawberries
- Imported nectarines
- Imported grapes
- Sweet bell peppers
- Domestic blueberries
- Kale and collard greens

CHAPTER 5

The Importance of Diet on Baby's Gene Expression

In the modern age, women are instructed to start eating a healthy diet once they find out they're pregnant. For our primitive ancestors, and those who continue to live a more traditional lifestyle, eating healthy starts much earlier. Native people prepare for pregnancy with special foods *at least* six months prior to the date of conception.

How Primitive People Prepare for Favorable Gene Expression

Weston A. Price observed these practices all over the world. He noted that "primitive peoples have carried out programs that will produce physically excellent babies. This they have achieved by a system of carefully planned nutritional programs for mothers-to-be. It is important to note that they begin this process of special feeding long before conception takes place, not leaving it, as is so generally done, until after the mother-to-be knows she is pregnant."

Often, members of the tribe would either go to great lengths to acquire these special foods or wait until the right foods were available before trying to conceive. Among the Masai, says Weston A. Price, "the girls were required to wait for marriage until the time of the year when the cows were on the rapidly growing young grass and to use the milk from these cows for a certain number of months before they could be married. In several agricultural tribes in Africa, the girls were fed on special foods for six months before marriage."

In Fiji, he photographed a tribal woman holding up a lobster-crab. The woman had "come a long distance to gather special foods needed for the production of a healthy child. These and many primitive people have understood the necessity for special foods before marriage, during gestation, during the nursing period and for rebuilding before the next pregnancy."

He also observed tribes going to great trouble to obtain iodine-rich plants. "In Africa I found many tribes gathering certain plants from swamps and marshes and streams, particularly the water hyacinth. These plants were dried and burned for their ashes which were put into the foods of mothers and growing children."

Throughout his travels, he observed primitives eating the organs of animals. Often they were reserved for women and children. "Among the Indians in the moose country near the Arctic circle, a larger percentage of the children were born in June than in any other month. This was accomplished, I was told, by both parents eating liberally of the thyroid glands of the male moose as they came down from the high mountain areas for the mating season, at which time the large protuberances carrying the thyroids under the throat were greatly enlarged."

What is even more fascinating is that these special practices are taking place amongst people who *already* eat diets nutritionally superior to our own. All of their foods are grown in rich soil. They have no contact with nutritionally deficient food whatsoever; every morsel they put in their mouths is healthy. Yet still they seek even higher quality foods in preparation for a baby.

They do this because they realize that certain foods taken prior to conception serve two purposes. It helps improve fertility, boosting a woman's chances of getting pregnant. And it offers babies and children the best chance of health and strength. Native people themselves didn't and don't know the science behind how certain nutrients set up a baby for a more favorable gene expression; the proof of their value is in thousands of years of experience. What we have learned through science they learned through time-tested observation.

Genetics Basics

Genes are instructions contained in our DNA, which is housed in our chromosomes. Humans have 46 chromosomes. Our parents each give us a random combination of 23 of their chromosomes to make up our 46. Inside are thousands of different genes that guide various aspects of our growth, development, and health. The Human Genome Project has estimated that humans have a total of between 20,000 to 25,000 genes. Most humans share the same genes—in fact, only about 1 percent of our genes differ. That works out to about 200 or so genes that differ between random people like you and me (siblings are obviously going to be more similar), yet that's enough to make us all pretty unique.

This is basic genetics. It starts to get really interesting when you look at gene expression. Not all of those thousands of genes contained in your 46 chromosomes will "turn on." A person can carry the gene for celiac disease, for example, and never actually show signs or symptoms. If that person passes down the gene to his or her offspring, that child may express the gene and exhibit celiac disease even though neither of the parents did.

Geneticists used to think that gene expression was the luck of the draw. This is still the prevalent notion among lay people. You hear people saying, "My mother had heart attacks, my father and grandparents had heart attacks, so I guess I'd better brace myself." But this view of genetics is naïve.

Epigenetics—"Above the Genome"

When most people think of making babies out of sperm and egg, they think the genes from the mom and dad equal baby. That's it. As far as genes are concerned, you get what you get. But this isn't the whole picture. Certain factors actually affect the way our genes *behave*. It's a phenomenon called epigenetics, which refers to the role that factors such as diet, stress, and environment play on gene behavior without actually altering the DNA sequence of the gene itself.

Randy Jirtle, of the Jirtle laboratory at Duke University, said that Epigenetics literally means "'above the genome.' So if you think, for example, of the genome as being like the hardware of a computer, the epigenome would be the software that tells the computer when to work, how to work, and how much."

Environmental factors such as stress, diet, and exposure to toxins like BPA (Bisphenol A), which is used in the manufacture of plastics and epoxy resins, all influence gene behavior through the combined effects of DNA methylation and histone modifications. Methyl groups—chemical tags of carbon and hydrogen that affix to the gene—shut down genes by attaching to them and inhibiting their functions. Other tags called histones also control gene expression. Together, these patterns influence the way the genome is expressed. This translates to an incredibly powerful idea: We are not slaves to our genes.

"A huge body of evidence now supports the notion that these diseases [heart disease and cancer] are linked to poor fetal growth followed by adequate or even an excess of food in childhood. While we are not doomed by our prenatal and early nutritional exposures, they do make us more vulnerable to disease," said David Barker, MD, PhD, professor of medicine at Oregon Health and Sciences University.

The implications of the epigenome are profound and far-reaching. With the power to control our gene expression we are ultimately responsible for our health. The decisions we make—like whether we choose to smoke, drink excessively, or eat a nutrient deficient diet—all play a role in whether we will end up with diseases like cancer later in life and even whether we will pass them down to our children. While at first that may seem like an unwanted a burden, it should also give us hope: We have the power to improve the lives of ourselves and our children.

Nutrition For Maximum Health

Mothers try to eat "healthy" to avoid a miscarriage, and to ensure that the baby develops without any serious deformities. But eating a nutrient-dense diet can also give our children the gift of strong, beautiful, and disease-free bodies.

Babies will grow with or without optimal nutrition, but certain nutrients can mean the difference between a high IQ or a low one, between chronic disease and health. The nutrition the baby receives while in the womb sets up the child for a lifetime of ills or easy sailing.

"We're showing that it's the maternal behavior that counts, not just the genetic baggage," says Moshe Szyf, PhD, who researches epigenetics and is a professor of Pharmacology and Therapeutics at McGill University in Montreal. "Behavior can clearly affect the chemistry of DNA."

Familiar nutrients like folate, B12, choline, betaine, methionine, and SAM-e (S-Adenosyl methionine) can rapidly alter gene expression, especially during early development when the epigenome is first being established. Foods rich in choline include liver and muscle meats, eggs, brussel sprouts, and dark chocolate. Liver, leafy greens, kombucha, nuts, and chicken all contain folate. There is no food source of SAM-e but certain nutrients are required for its production. To produce SAM-e we must eat foods rich in Vitamin B12 and folate and avoid drugs and excessive amounts of alcohol.

If, like our primitive ancestors, we make every effort to avoid harmful substances, maintain a low stress level, and include these special nutrients during and before pregnancy, we can save our children from expressing undesirable genes.

CHAPTER 6

Exercise During and After Pregnancy

The American College of Obstetricians and Gynecologists give pregnant women very conservative recommendations for exercise during pregnancy. As a result of these recommendations and decades of wrong-headed thinking, women worry that strenuous activity will damage the baby. Many researchers, however, including Dr. James F. Clapp—a pioneer in the field of medicine and exercise physiology—say that exercising while pregnant is not only safe but necessary for the maintenance of good health.

Myths

While it is true that pregnant women need to follow guidelines while exercising, many of the concerns are myths. For example:

1. Abdominal exercises of any kind should be avoided after the first trimester.
2. Pregnant women should refrain from any supine exercise (lying on the back) after the first trimester.
3. Running and bouncing exercises are not safe for the fetus.
4. Bouncing exercises can weaken the pelvic floor.
5. Exercising longer than 20 minutes at a time will overheat the baby and take needed oxygen and nutrients away from the placenta.

Pregnant women are a whole lot stronger than we are led to believe, or at least they can be. Dr. Clapp has argued that a pregnant woman's body is as well prepared for the demands of strenuous exercise as that of an athlete. A pregnant woman has expanded blood volume, larger heart chambers, greater blood volume per heartbeat, and faster transfer of oxygen to tissues. Athletes also exhibit these differences. Fit women are able to adjust to pregnancy faster than women who don't exercise because their bodies are already halfway there. Again, care must be taken to ensure that the mother and baby stay safe—adjustments must be made and rest periods taken—but exercise while pregnant is safe, natural, and offers myriad benefits to mother and baby.

Benefits to the Mother

- **Reduces aches and pains**—Exercise improves posture by strengthening the back and abs. These muscles are essential for comfortably carrying around a 10 pound-or-more tummy.

- **Improves circulation**—Improved circulation confers several benefits: It can help prevent constipation and cramps; and improved blood flow reduces the swelling in legs that causes varicose veins.

- **Prevents wear and tear on the joints**—Exercise helps to stabilize joints and offsets the effect of the pregnancy hormone relaxin, which relaxes the ligaments that support the joints.

- **Boosts immune system**—Dr. Clapp's research team observed that the incidence of colds, flu, sinusitis, and bronchitis is lower in exercisers.

- **Lowers gestational diabetes risk by 27 percent**—Exercise helps to keep blood sugar even.

- **Faster recovery**—Maintaining a high level of fitness helps moms get back to a regular exercise routine more quickly than non-exercising moms; the body remains toned and proper weight is maintained.

- **Reduces mood swings and stress**—Exercise boosts the serotonin and endorphins that make us feel happier.

- **Reduces fatigue**—Pregnant women often feel tired in the first and third trimesters, making it hard to get moving. But make the effort: Active pregnant women have more energy in general and they have a higher tolerance for the stresses of pregnancy and infant care.

- **Improves sleep**—Pregnant women who keep up an exercise routine often report better quality sleep. However, exercising too close to bedtime can contribute to insomnia.

- **Reduces morning sickness**—While feeling nauseous can make it difficult to exercise, many women report reduced nausea after a workout.

- **Keeps weight in check**—Clapp showed that women who exercise all the way through the end of their pregnancy gain, on average, 8 pounds less than their sedentary counterparts.

- **Improves body image**—Being fit helps a woman feel better about herself—especially when that big belly is making her feel a little less than sexy.

- **Speeds and eases delivery**—Having a baby requires strength and stamina. What better way to prepare for this than by being strong and cardiovascularly fit? Studies have also shown that pregnant women who exercise need fewer painkillers, probably because their endorphins (natural painkillers) are higher.

- **Trains a better athlete**—Clapp found that women who train all the way through their pregnancies "increase their maximum aerobic capacity by 5 to 10 percent." This is true despite the fact that their pregnancy training levels were actually lower during pregnancy than before pregnancy.

- **Produces smaller babies at birth**—Babies of exercising moms are not as fat but just as long and robust as the heavier babies born to mothers who don't exercise.

Benefits to the Baby

- **Leaner children**—These babies will be leaner all the way up to their fifth birthday, assuming their diets are packed with the right nutrients, and long after that if they continue to eat properly and exercise.

- **Stronger fetal cardiovascular system**—Researchers from the Kansas City University of Medicine and Biosciences found that the fetus is more than just a passive observer of mother's exercise routine. Fetuses of mothers who exercise have stronger hearts, much like the exerciser herself.

- **Improved tolerance to the stress of delivery**—Studies have shown that babies born to exercising moms experience less stress at the time of delivery.

- **Fewer infant problems**—The newborns of exercising mothers are reported to have less colic, sleep through the night, and are easier to care for in general.

♦ **Faster growing placenta**—This means more nutrients and oxygen for the baby. If no other reason gets you moving, this one should!

Types of Exercise for the Pregnant Woman

The Best Type of Exercise During Pregnancy

Any kind of weight-bearing exercise offers the most benefits to a pregnant woman and her baby. While walking, stretching, and yoga are all highly beneficial, none of them have the added benefit of building muscle and improving the aerobic endurance that will be necessary during delivery. To obtain the most benefits, either lift weights, climb hills, do interval sprints, or any other exercise that challenges the muscles. While yoga can offer muscle building benefits if poses are held for long enough periods of time, I have found most prenatal yoga classes to be too easy on mothers-to-be.

When I was pregnant with Evelyn, my summer exercise of choice was hiking in the Santa Cruz Mountains. I did this several times a week. It was my time to disconnect from the busy modern world and reconnect with nature. Not only did it offer me time for reflection, it strengthened my muscles and improved my stamina. This preparation helped me stay strong from the beginning, then recover quickly. After Evelyn was born, I continued to hike with her in my backpack until she was almost three.

Should You Avoid Extreme Sports?

I am a snowboarder and I learned of my second pregnancy right after I bought my season pass. After reading up on the subject, I decided that as long as I listened to my body—drank plenty of water, took breaks as needed, stayed off the big jumps, that sort of thing—I'd probably be fine in early pregnancy. The first time I went up while pregnant I was a little nervous, but I quickly realized that downhill riding was safe. I've been snowboarding for 16 years and am a very controlled rider. Once I got to 16 weeks pregnant, however, I was done. At that point I could feel the baby kick and knew that if I could feel her, she could feel a hard impact.

Researchers who advocate exercise through pregnancy believe that even a sport as challenging as mountain climbing can be continued as long as ropes are used. But I agree with the American College of Obstetricians and Gynecologists that a few sports should be avoided: Scuba diving, due to the dangers of decompression, and contact sports. They also recommend avoiding downhill snow sports, but I think it's fine if you are experienced, take precautions, and stop at 16 weeks, when the fetus becomes susceptible to injury through the abdomen.

A Pregnant Woman's Center of Gravity

Here's another Western myth: Pregnant women have horrible balance and are hopelessly clumsy because their center of gravity is off. They can't do most yoga poses because they'll fall over like a toddler; if they try to ride a bike, they'll topple over sideways; if they walk on uneven surfaces they might trip; if they dance they will bump into people; and if any random object gets under their feet, they'll fall down and break a bone.

None of this needs to happen. For one thing, we have time to get used to our new bodies; it's not like we wake up one morning with a ten-pound ball in our tummies. The change is gradual and we learn to maneuver, and keeping active during pregnancy is a great way to make sure to maintain good balance.

While traveling in Colombia, I noticed that even pregnant women ride bikes. It seemed crazy to me when I saw it. But they weren't wobbly or fearful. That's when I began to think that maybe the idea that pregnant women are clumsy is cultural. Maybe we're not meant to be this way at all. With this pregnancy I've had the opportunity to try it out myself.

One day, when I was six months pregnant, I needed to go to the store, but didn't have a car available. So I hopped on my bike to get where I needed to go. To my surprise, it wasn't any different than it had been before! My balance wasn't off, I wasn't wobbly, and it was a great pleasure. I've continued to enjoy riding my bike on park paths throughout my pregnancy. I had almost the same epiphany when I found myself perfectly stable in my yoga class at six months pregnant. I had expected balancing poses to be a thing of the past, but I didn't find them difficult at all!

The ability to balance, of course, will depend on previous experience. While pregnancy shouldn't prevent women from carrying on with life as normal, now may not be the time to start riding a bike if you never have or haven't in years. Nor would it be the time to start experimenting with balancing poses.

Running and Jumping Exercises During Pregnancy

In the past, it was assumed that running and jumping were dangerous to the fetus and to the pelvic floor. However, many researchers and long-time runners like Paula Radcliffe and Kara Goucher have proven this to be yet another old wives' tale.

Running and jumping are perfectly safe for both women with a previous high fitness level and those just starting out. A beginner won't be finishing marathons at 39 weeks, like Amber Miller did. But the natural bouncing up and down that comes with running is not going to harm the baby. As with any strenuous exercise, however, pregnant women should always get plenty of rest, drink lots of water, and take it slowly.

How Much Exercise

Our hormones help us to adjust to varying levels of activity, but we don't have any that help us adjust to none at all. Throughout history, humans have been active for much of each day. Inactivity has no place in the history of human evolution and, hence, we have not adapted to sedentary lifestyles.

In addition to low bone density, poor circulation, weaker blood vessels and the countless other side effects of inactivity, being sedentary also causes a disruption in hormone balance. Exercising triggers insulin to drop. If we don't exercise, insulin can stay elevated. Chronically elevated insulin leads to hormonal imbalances that are bad for baby's genes and for mom's well-being.

The actual amount of exercise that will be beneficial is going to vary according to your individual fitness level—women who are just starting out will do less and women who've been exercising for a while will be able to do more—but to obtain the benefits seen in most studies, at least three hours a week of moderate to strenuous exercise must be maintained throughout the pregnancy. Beyond that, you should avoid sitting for extended periods of time, and move as much as you can during the day.

Warnings

As a general rule, rest when you feel fatigued and stop if you feel dizzy. When we're not pregnant we can afford to push our limits. Once you're pregnant, you must go easy, which can mean checking your ego at the gym door. (In other words, save the weightlifting championship for next year.) Never push yourself to the point of exhaustion. It's fine if you do it once or twice as you determine your personal limits, but once you do, stay within a comfortable range. As you progress, you'll get stronger and your stamina will increase. What I have found with my own pregnancies is that my body knows best. I know when I'm fatigued. I know when I'm uncomfortable. I know when I'm pushing it too far.

The standard recommendation for women is to keep the heart rate under 140 beats per minute while exercising. Fit pregnant women will rarely get their hearts over that anyway because the body has become more efficient at pumping blood. As long as you stay within a comfortable range you should be fine. There are, however, conditions that generally preclude exercise during pregnancy.

Contraindications

- If you are extremely under- or overweight
- If fetal growth is poor
- If you experience early pregnancy bleeding
- If you have a history of three or more miscarriages

Guidelines for the pregnant exerciser:

- Be prepared. Rising altitude or increases in heat or cold can affect your expectations. When I was four months pregnant with Evelyn, I went from my sea level home in California to visit family in Colorado. I set out on a three-mile hike without even thinking about the new conditions. The altitude was 6000 feet higher than in California, and the temperature was 100 degrees (it was August). The hike was miserable. The baby was fine, and so was I, but I spent the whole time worrying about our health rather than enjoying my time in nature.
- If exercise hurts, stop.
- When tired, take a break.
- If experiencing abnormal daytime fatigue, ease up on the routine.
- Be flexible with the routine, duration, and type of exercise. Boredom or overtraining may result if you do the same things day after day.
- Sleep more. A pregnant woman should try to get one extra hour of rest for every hour of exercise.
- In mid-to-late pregnancy, if the baby doesn't move two to three times within 30 minutes of exercising, the fetus is experiencing undue stress. Ease up on the routine next time.

Exercising After Pregnancy

The great thing about staying fit during pregnancy is that you can begin exercising much sooner after the baby is born. Most fit women can start within the first couple of weeks after delivery. Just remember: You will be exhausted, busy, and recovering from childbirth, so take it easy at first. If you stay fit, however, it's nice to know you won't be down for months. Eating well and getting rest will also make your workouts easier once you're ready. The exercises should be gentle at first; you don't want to break down muscle tissue while your body is working hard to rebuild it. And focus first on realignment and balance—the number one priority for the postpartum woman.

Alignment

As the fetus grows and the center of gravity shifts, the pelvis tips forward and the pubic bone moves back. The chest responds by tipping forward, the neck tilts down and forward, and the abdominal muscles stretch so much that they become virtually worthless for lower back support. Before we get back to our regular exercise routine, we need to first correct these issues of misalignment.

Challenges to Alignment

- **Sitting too much**—Not only do most of our jobs demand that we sit for eight-or-more hours a day, but the majority of us drive everywhere we go. Make a conscious effort to get up off your chair and move, whether you're pregnant or not. A standing desk is a smart option. If that isn't possible, stand up every hour or two and walk around the office or your house.

- **Slouching**—Not only do we sit too much but we sit without lower back support. This causes slouching. If you don't have an ergonomic chair or driver's seat, add a small pillow to prop the lower back.

- **Tipping the pelvis back while standing**—Pregnant women often try to compensate for a bigger belly by tipping the pelvis back. This can cause back pain and, if you're lifting weights or even just taking a walk, it can cause injury. When standing, keep your pelvis right over your heels and your shoulders over your hips. You should be able to comfortably lift your toes off the floor without losing your balance.

- **Waddling**—Pregnant women don't have to walk like a duck. When they do, it's a sign of bad alignment. Aim for straight posture, feet facing forward, not out, and arms swinging comfortably at our your sides.

For specific alignment exercises, see chapters 10 and 13.

Gentle Postpartum Exercises

If a mother starts with gentle exercises, she can begin practicing them the day after the baby is born. These can help get her ready for the real thing.

Start with light abdominal tensions, breathing exercises, Kegels (pelvic floor exercises), and stretches. All of these can be done in bed when baby is sleeping. As strength builds, additional regular exercise may be added, beginning with walking.

- **All in one: deep breathing, abdominal muscles, and Kegel**—Inhale slowly and deeply through the nose, expanding only the belly. As you exhale gently draw your abdominal muscles in as you simultaneously tense the muscles of the pelvic floor. Slowly release and repeat. This exercise prepares the abdominals and pelvic floor muscles for more advanced abdominal exercises (see chapter 13).

- **Buttocks squeeze**—Lie on your back with knees bent and the small of the back flat against the bed or on the floor. Inhale deeply. As you exhale, squeeze your buttocks without lifting your hips. Slowly release and repeat. This will help improve circulation and prepare you for walking.

- **Stretches**—If you find yourself in bed a lot in the first few days following birth, periodically stretch your arms and legs out, arch your back, reach your arms toward your toes, and roll your wrists and ankles. All of these movements will improve circulation.

- **Walking**—Within two or three days, you should start walking short distances—slowly and with plenty of rest periods.

PART II

The Collagen Connection

Genetics is often blamed for stretch marks, cellulite, varicose veins, sagging breasts and bottoms, wrinkles and jowls. The real villain responsible for these post-baby miseries is weak connective tissue, which most American women have thanks to all the damaging fats, sugars, and inflammatory chemicals in our diet. In the next six chapters, I will describe the consequences of weak connective tissue and how to strengthen it so that you can be proud of your body before and after you have a baby.

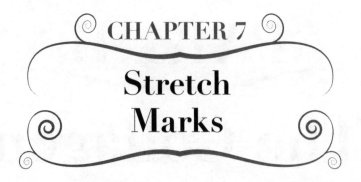

CHAPTER 7

Stretch Marks

Stretch marks affect between 70 and 90 percent of pregnant women. So chances are good that you are going to get them. For many of us, the thought of going through life scarred by these shiny white marks is disturbing, but we want children so we make the sacrifice. Then we make up cute phrases for them, like "beautiful reminders of carrying a child" or the "exclusive symbol of the special sect called mothers."

If you already have stretch marks from a previous pregnancy, I'm not trying to make you feel bad. I have my share of scars too. But it is important to realize that they are not "the beauty marks of a mother." Rather they are the consequence of malnutrition, inflammation, and hormonal imbalance. By seeing stretch marks for what they are, we can strive to take better care of ourselves.

What are Stretch Marks?

Most people believe these marks are an inevitable consequence of the skin stretching during pregnancy. The idea is intuitive and, as ubiquitous as stretch marks are, it seems to follow. But think about it for a moment. If this were true, wouldn't the belly of every postpartum woman exhibit stretch marks? In fact, while every pregnant belly expands, there are women who do not end up with those telltale marks. Furthermore, it's not just pregnant women who get stretch marks; so do young girls going through puberty, weightlifters, and people who gain weight rapidly—and their skin is not stretching as dramatically as a pregnant woman's does. This tells us that something besides stretching must be at work here.

The situation simply isn't as simple as *skin stretches, marks appear.* Striae, or stretch marks, are scars which form on the second layer of the skin (the dermis), just beneath the outer layer (epidermis). They are not so much marks formed by stretching skin as actual wounds from torn and damaged tissue. These tear wounds start deep, in the dermis, then rise to epidermis, where they become visible to the naked eye. You may have tried repairing and preventing stretch marks with creams with no luck. That's because the solution must come from within. To understand why, let's first talk about your skin and the causes of tearing.

The Layers of the Skin

- **The epidermis** is a transparent layer of dead skin cells that provides waterproofing and pigment.

- **The dermis** is the middle or second layer of the skin and contains a corrugated layer of blood vessels, nerves, hair follicles, and sweat glands. The dermis is primarily composed of connective tissue containing collagen and elastin (both naturally occurring proteins). These woven tissues provide elasticity and flexibility, cushioning the body from stress and strain (the dermis is why your skin doesn't become marked with depressions and pinches every time it's touched).

- **The sub-dermis** anchors the skin with a connective layer of fat, providing fat storage and insulation.

Damage to Connective Tissue

When the skin stretches, the tissue in the dermis layer can break down and become compromised, resulting in a wound. Damage to tissues leads to blood vessel dilation (these are the early stage red or purplish lines). Later, as the body tries to heal itself from the breaks in the top epithelial cells, cells begin dividing to fill in the gap. If the damage was deep enough, the cells produce a fibrous mass (a scar) to heal the wound. In this case the melanin production will cease and the skin will be left with white hypopigmented scars—those shiny, white stretch marks that never go away.

Who Gets Stretch Marks?

Stretch marks can appear on pregnant women, pubescent teens, body builders, women who take birth control pills, and people who gain or lose weight rapidly. They can appear on a body of any size, on people of every color, and on men and women, though more often on women.

In a study of 324 maternal test subjects, researchers found that women of low maternal age are more susceptible to severe stretch marks, "a finding not found in women over 30 years of age." The same study also found that women who gain in excess of 33 pounds during pregnancy, or whose maternal body mass index was greater than 26, were at higher risk.

Location

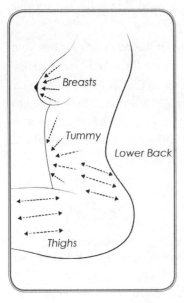

- During pregnancy, stretch marks usually appear on the belly, but they may appear anywhere if the mother experiences significant weight gain.

- Pubescent teens will see stretch marks on the hips and buttocks.

- During periods of rapid weight gain, stretch marks can appear almost anywhere, but typically on parts of the body with a greater body fat percentage (e.g., thighs, buttocks, hips, calves, or arms).

- Bodybuilders sometimes develop stretch marks at the top of the pectoral muscles and across the shoulders.

The Cause: Weak Collagen

Stretching alone is not enough to cause stretch marks. The skin is actually quite elastic and is designed to stretch. Stretch marks are an indication that the skin is weak and cannot withstand the normal changes that pregnant women must undergo.

Stretch marks occur when the connective tissue in the dermal layer of the skin degrades. When that tissue is thinned or dry, it will tear just like a dry rubber band. But what causes the degradation of connective tissue in the first place? Why does it thin and become dry? There are many contributing factors. These include the poor diet of our mothers while we were in utero, life-long and present nutrient deficiencies, cellular dehydration, imbalance of hormones, and poor circulation. All of these factors influence the production of collagen, which provides strength and thickness to our skin and joints.

Collagen makes up about 75 percent of the weight of the skin. It is the most extensive structural protein in the body. Collagen is what cushions and strengthens the joints and what unites the cells in our organs and skin, imparting strength and flexibility to the whole body. Strong collagen is important both for beauty and for functionality. When it is weak, we experience everything from joint injuries to sagging jowls, butts, and breasts; from wrinkles to cellulite; from stretch marks to thin veins.

When the skin is healthy, it will stretch without damage. In the case of the dramatic but gradual stretching that occurs during pregnancy, the skin will make new collagen to strengthen the collagen layers as they thin out, enabling the skin to safely stretch more and more. That's because the connective tissue is constantly being reinforced with more collagen fibers. It can do this as long as it has the building blocks it needs to make new elastic fibers.

Stretch marks and other symptoms of weak connective tissue, like joint injuries, are becoming very common in our modern world. And while most of us think the problem is due to the expansion of the skin, running too much, or aging, the real problem is the shifts in nutrition over the last century. The building blocks of collagen come from the nutrition in foods that most of us rarely eat. The problem starts with the bad diets of our mothers and grandmothers, continues with inactivity and a diet deficient in essential nutrients, and then progresses with the ensuing imbalance of hormones.

The Five Factors Contributing to Weak Collagen:

+ **Genetics**
+ **Nutritional deficiencies**
+ **High glucocorticoid hormones**
+ **Dehydration**
+ **Poor circulation**

Genes

Some women are lucky: They had mothers and grandmothers who ate the right foods while they were pregnant, resulting in strong collagen-forming cells, which they then passed down to their children. Eating a diet that promotes collagen production can program the genes to be collagen-producing machines. The benefits are even greater when mothers feed their children the same nutritious diet in early childhood.

If you are endowed with strong collagen, these layers can last a long time. If that's you, you may avoid most of the problems associated with weak collagen (like joint problems and wrinkles) well into old age. However, if you have adopted a nutrient-deficient Standard American Diet (the acronyn, appropriately, is SAD), even great genes won't save you. Remember, genes are not set in stone; their expression changes with the quality of your diet.

Nutritional Deficiencies

Nutrients such as protein, Vitamin C, and zinc are critical for collagen synthesis. Without them, stretch marks will likely result during pregnancy.

To produce collagen, you have to eat protein. But in order to synthesize that protein into collagen fibers, you need Vitamin C. If you're undergoing any significant skin stretching, as you do during pregnancy, you'll also need zinc, to help heal the wounds as they form; plenty of broth from the connective tissue of animals, for both their collagen and their water-attracting, collagen-seeking molecules (called *glycosaminoglycans*); and magnesium, to maintain the balanced hormones necessary for strong collagen. If our diets aren't nutrient-dense, then our skin will not have what it needs to rebound from the stretching of the belly (or any other part of the body).

Glucocorticoids

Recent research on stretch marks has centered around hormones, particularly the glucocorticoid hormones (including cortisol). These are thought to play a role in the development of stretch marks by preventing the fibroblasts (the cell in the connective tissue which synthesizes collagen) from forming new collagen. This is a critical function of skin repair, particularly during the process of stretching. When collagen is damaged, new fibers must be formed to keep the skin elastic and healthy.

Glucocorticoids are adrenal hormones that are released in response to stress. They are known to substantially increase during pregnancy, adolescence, obesity, and during intense periods of weight lifting. Other hormones increase during these times as well, but research points to glucocorticoids because they have been observed to prevent the fibroblasts from repairing and regenerating the collagen and elastin fiber network. What researchers have yet to determine is why some women get stretch marks while pregnant and some don't, at what point glucocorticoid levels become detrimental to collagen synthesis, and how those hormone levels can be controlled.

These are some of the questions that scientists are currently investigating. I imagine research will eventually lead to a drug that at-risk individuals can take to lower glucocorticoids, thus preventing stretch marks. A treatment like this, of course, will only be a temporary solution for a deeper problem contributing to the degradation of collagen.

While doctors search for the next miracle drug, you can take action to lower glucocorticoids by reducing stress and avoiding low blood sugar and insulin resistance. Low blood sugar levels and insulin resistance cause the adrenal glands to release cortisol. Maintaining even blood sugar levels by avoiding excess fructose (including high fructose corn syrup in processed foods) and sugar, and by including saturated fat will help to keep corticosteroids under control.

Dehydration

Hydration also plays a big role in skin health. If the cells of the skin are dried out, the elasticity will be compromised. Most people don't drink enough water and don't eat enough natural fats to keep the body well hydrated. Their importance, however, cannot be overstated. This is what the Linus Pauling Institute has to say about Transepidermal Water Loss (TEWL):

> *"Dry skin can be caused by many factors, but it is usually accompanied by changes in the epidermal barrier and increased TEWL (more water lost to the environment). Intrinsic changes in the lipid barrier or NMF of the stratum corneum can disrupt the barrier and cause water loss. This can stem from simple chemical exposures, such as washing with detergents, or from more complex nutritional deficiencies, such as a lack of essential fatty acids. However, dry skin can also be an effect of atmospheric conditions or exposures. Changes in temperature, airflow, and humidity can pull water away from the skin and reduce barrier integrity. If left untreated, dry skin is often predisposed to insults from other sources, leading to cycles of cell damage and inflammation that perpetuate the condition."*

Water, saturated fat, and cholesterol are all hydrating on a cellular level. The three act together as the bonding adhesives in the cell membrane. The fats need to be eaten and carried to each cell of the body. Eating fat is also necessary for absorption of the fat-soluble Vitamins A, D, and E, all of which prevent skin from drying out. Following a "heart healthy" diet by eliminating saturated fat and dietary cholesterol and replacing them with polyunsaturated fats (PUFAs) can actually weaken cells.

Poor Circulation

Poor circulation is not a proven cause of stretch marks. However, good circulation is critical to the delivery of nutrients to all our cells. When the skin expands, the connective tissues, which are damaged at this time, need to be repaired. Hence more nutrients need to be delivered. Additionally, when circulation is poor, the skin is the first to suffer. The organs of the body take priority over the skin, so when circulation is poor, skin health is sacrificed in order to keep the rest of the body well.

While poor circulation can be caused by serious health conditions such as hypothyroidism, arteriosclerosis, and venous thrombosis, for most of us poor circulation can be improved by making a few lifestyle changes, exercise being chief among them. Nutrients are carried to our cells by our blood and the single best way to get blood flowing is to exercise.

Ethnicity

People of color are often believed to have less of a problem with stretch marks. Yet in a survey by the department of dermatology at Sanford University School of Medicine, Dr. Alexa B. Kimball said that nearly 80 percent of American women of color (African-American, Hispanic, Southeast Asian, among others) said they had stretch marks. In this survey, researchers sampled 161 women who had given birth.

Climate

People in humid climates have been shown to have less of a problem with hydration on the epidermis. However, the epidermis acts as a waterproof shield. Providing the epidermis with moisture either through humidity or body lotion does little to hydrate the deeper layers of the skin. The one benefit that a humid climate (or body lotion) can provide is the reduction of transepidermal water loss. Dry climates can dry out even healthy skin. While your skin may indeed benefit by spending nine months in the Caribbean (and a Caribbean pregnancy would definitely rock!), that's not practical for most of us. What is available to everyone is a healthy Primal diet.

Prevention

Eating a highly nutritious diet is the single best preventative medicine. Sure, there are women who eat horribly throughout their lives and pregnancies and still manage to slip through without a mark. But they are the exception, not the rule. The only way to prevent stretch marks while pregnant is to take good care of yourself. I will go over specific dietary and lifestyle strategies in chapter 13. But for improving connective tissue, the basics include:

- Eating broths made from the bones and connective tissues of other animals
- Eating greens for minerals
- Eating citrus for Vitamin C and bioflavonoids
- Eating fish and butter for cell building fats
- Exercising every day to carry nutrients to the skin
- Keeping stress low

Circulation

Poor circulation is very common, and serious conditions, like hypothyroidism, can cause it. But there are many simple steps we can take to improve the problem right now.

- **Exercise** carries nutrients to the cells by increasing blood flow.
- **Massage** helps to stimulate the flow of blood and lymph, moving toxins out and nutrients in.
- **Dry skin brushing** stimulates circulation directly to the skin.
- **Gingko Biloba**, an herb, has been used for centuries to increase circulation to the brain and other parts of the body.
- **Calendula** and other herbs help improve circulation topically.
- **Cayenne pepper, ginger, and garlic** can be eaten to improve blood flow.
- **Cigarettes** impair blood flow throughout the body and should be avoided. (This is pretty obvious if you're pregnant. If you're not pregnant yet, stop now to improve all-over health, as well as the likelihood of avoiding stretch marks).
- **Low blood sugar** levels affect circulation to the extremities, including the skin.

How to do Dry Skin Brushing

Dry skin brushing helps to prevent stretch marks by improving circulation to the skin and encouraging new skin cell growth. As old cells are sloughed off, new ones are encouraged to grow. Dry skin brushing has the added benefit of detoxifying the lymph. If stretch marks are already present, brushing should be avoided as the skin is delicate and the loofa can cause irritation.

A loofa sponge can be picked up at the health food store for just a few bucks. Loofa is a natural hard fiber that is particularly efficient at sloughing off old skin cells and encouraging circulation. Methods vary but Dr. Bruce Berkowsky, author of the "Vital Chi Skin-Brushing System," recommends small circular movements starting at the underarms and groin and moving towards the heart. The legs should come last, with the movements also moving towards the heart.

Topical Creams

Some expensive topical creams containing collagen-building materials such as Vitamin C have been shown to be useful in hydrating the epidermis. But remember: Stretch marks start from below the epidermis and work their way out. Building collagen from within is a more effective way to strengthen and rebuild collagen fibers.

Less expensive creams, including cocoa butter and other oils, are as effective as a placebo. Research is ongoing, however, with preparations utilizing everything from zinc to special hormone delivery systems. There are some preparations that pregnant women should avoid. Synthetic Vitamin A can cause birth defects. Natural forms of Vitamin A can be found in butter and fish oil, but you'd have to be either single or crazy to lather up with the scents of fish and butter. Many anti-wrinkle creams and anti-stretch mark creams contain the nutrients your skin needs to produce collagen, but be very careful: Many contain dangerous chemicals. For a searchable database of cosmetic ingredients, visit the website of the Environmental Working Group (http://www.ewg.org/).

Reversal

Once the red lines of stretch marks appear, you have already reached the danger zone; the skin is wounded and scars will take their place. Good nutrition can help to minimize the impact of these scars and can even reduce the appearance of old scars to some degree but, in general, we are stuck with our scars forever. I don't know about you, but my knees are still covered with skateboarding and bicycle accident scars from childhood.

I had imbalanced hormones throughout my teens and twenties and, during puberty, I developed stretch marks on my hips. However, after going Paleo before my first pregnancy, I balanced my hormones by switching to a nutrient-dense diet and did not get them again. Once the factors which predispose us to stretch marks change, so does our susceptibility. The stretch marks I developed in my teens are still there, of course, but all is not lost. While stretch marks will never totally disappear, they can become next to invisible by following a nutrient-dense Primal diet and taking care of the skin.

- **Keep weight down.** Stretch marks are indented lines that lack the plumpness of normal skin. These white depressions can widen when we gain weight, making them almost glisten. When weight is down, each stretch mark line will be so thin as to be barely visible.

- **Keep skin hydrated from within**. When the skin itself is plump, scars look filled in and are less visible. Just as wrinkles are more visible when the skin is dehydrated, so are scars and stretch marks.

- **Hydrate skin from without**. Undoubtedly, stretch marks are less visible when the skin is moist. Apply lotion or coconut oil to temporarily mask the problem.

- **Use self-tanner**. Tanning will not help the stretch marks to blend in with the rest of the skin since the mark does not produce melanin (skin pigment). In fact, tanning can make them even more unsightly by increasing the contrast between the healthy and scarred skin. But a self-tanner can help, adding just enough color back to the white scar.

Cosmetic Procedures

While it is ideal to become pro-active about your health and fight stretch marks from within, once the damage is done, it is done. A nutritious diet can help to improve scars but not to heal them completely. Women with extensive stretch marks can feel disfigured when their buttocks, breasts, and bellies are covered in white or red lines. For most of us, the damage is not severe enough to consider expensive procedures, but if you had a baby before learning of the dietary principles set forth in this book your only option—other than choosing to ignore them—may be modern technology. One of the newest treatments is fractional laser therapy. I do not know how remarkable or unremarkable this treatment is; most of the literature is written by people selling it. But the claim is that the laser can reduce, and even eliminate, the appearance of stretch marks (and scars) by removing the fibrous mass and encouraging the production of melanin.

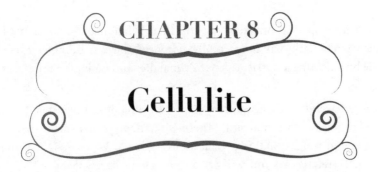

CHAPTER 8

Cellulite

With a little bit of effort, just about anybody can look good with clothes on—corsets hold in the belly, tight jeans hold up the butt, and most pants will hide the lumps—but looking good naked requires attention to what lies beneath your skin. Cellulite is, like so many other symptoms, a sign of degeneration. Ignoring degeneration is not a great strategy for health. If you have cellulite, and you're reading this book to learn how to improve it, you are doing yourself a greater service than you probably realize. The same weakened connective tissue that's behind cellulite is also the cause of joint and artery degradation. So paying attention to those little lumps on your thighs just might save you from heart attacks and hip replacements down the road.

Myths About Cellulite

+ **Cellulite is a Disease**. It is not, in itself, a disease. It is a symptom that can indicate future susceptibility to disease.

+ **Cellulite is Fat**. It is not "fat," per se. It is merely the way in which fat is displayed on some women's bodies.

+ **Skinny girls don't get cellulite**. Thin women can have just as many dimples on their thighs as woman twice their weight.

+ **Sugar is the cause of cellulite**. Many women on low carb diets still struggle with cellulite.

+ **Losing weight will lose the cellulite**. Losing weight does little to alleviate cellulite.

+ **Cellulite happens to all women at some point**. This is becoming more and more true as our diets become less and less adequate, but, thankfully, we can prevent cellulite. It does not have to be a part of aging.

- **Cellulite is just a cosmetic problem**. Absolutely not true. Cellulite is a symptom of a much deeper problem.

- **Cellulite is genetic and I can't change my genes**. This is the old way of thinking about genetics. As we have already seen, we can influence our genes by choices we make throughout our lives.

Anatomy of Cellulite

Cellulite is the pitted, dimply skin that looks a little like the surface of an orange peel. Contrary to what you might think, it isn't fat. Every human body has a layer of fat on their bodies, which the dermis layer of skin is meant to conceal. Cellulite appears when subcutaneous herniated fat starts to bulge through the connective tissues of the dermis. That's why it shows up as little bulges and dimples.

Cellulite is generally located on the buttocks and thighs and sometimes makes an appearance on the abdomen and arms. It is estimated that 80-90 percent of women have it. Most of the time it develops during puberty or pregnancy, and with age.

Why Men Don't Have Cellulite

Cellulite is almost exclusively found on women because it is female hormones that cause the slight differences in skin structure (men who get cellulite generally have feminizing hormonal problems). Men have the advantage of thicker epidermis and dermis layers around the buttocks and thighs, as well as a thinner first fat layer (subdermal fat). More significantly, their subdermal fat is arranged in polygonal units separated by crisscrossing connective tissue. It is this crisscrossing that keeps the subdermal fat from pushing through the skin. Women's subdermal fat cells, on the other hand, line up in vertical columns and can fit larger quantities of fat inside the pocket with less of a connective tissue covering.

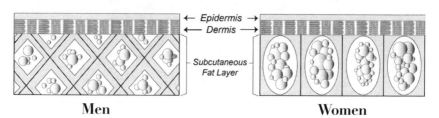

Men	Women

← Epidermis →
← Dermis →
Subcutaneous Fat Layer

This is not to say that a woman's skin *has* to exhibit cellulite. Rather, it's that if the conditions are ripe—i.e., connective tissue is thin, weak, and dry—chances are good that cellulite will occur.

Losing Weight Offers Minimal Relief

The reason why losing weight does little to conceal cellulite is because of the structure of the skin. The fat that is lost through diet and exercise is our normal fat. Normal fat is tucked nicely behind a solid layer of fascia and cannot bulge through the skin. The thin layer of subdermal fat is not lost during normal weight loss and will continue to bulge through the dermis's connective tissue (those unsightly lumps). Losing weight can offer a little relief by taking some of the pressure off of the layers, but usually it is not enough to eliminate cellulite.

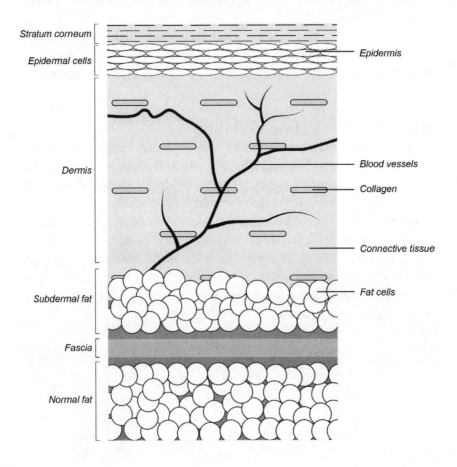

Experts Recognize Three Distinct Stages of Cellulite:

1. Since cellulite starts below the dermal layer, a person who is starting to develop cellulite won't be aware that it's happening. This is the stage when the dermis is just starting to lose its elasticity. Nutrients aren't being delivered to the dermis as efficiently as they should be. As with any condition, it takes time before the body actually exhibits symptoms. First the body starts to break down from underneath, then clues begin to surface.

2. Once the dermis is well on its way to deterioration, the skin might exhibit small patches of lumpiness, and may appear a little dry and less taut than it used to. When the skin is pinched, the cottage cheese appearance will be apparent. At this stage, women like to avoid sitting cross-legged.

3. Advanced cellulite can be seen without pinching the skin. Quite a bit of deterioration has occurred at this point; lack of firmness is apparent and affected areas may be bumpy to the touch.

Why Do Only Some Women Have Cellulite?

It's not fair, right? Even if you eat well and exercise, you can still be plagued with cellulite. But are all women doomed to suffer this dreaded blight? No, they're not! While a woman's anatomy, in general, offers the right conditions for cellulite to develop, it is not *caused* by this anatomy. It is caused by something else.

Cellulite appears when just the right combination of factors are present. One of those factors might be genetics, as in the lack of strong connective tissue in the genes. Others include hormonal imbalances and toxins that degrade tissues. Cellulite makes a greater appearance in heavier women and in women who are inactive. But the most common factor today is the lack of nutrition and the abundance of processed foods and sugar in our diets. Without proper nutrition, our connective tissue will break down, our hormones will be imbalanced, toxins will not freely flush out of our bodies, and dehydration will occur.

Cellulite is a sign of aging, much like wrinkles and sagging skin, but there are other reasons it occurs, from imbalanced hormones in adolescence to inadequate nutrition in early adulthood. For pregnant women, it happens when the undernourished mother turns over nutrients to the fetus.

The three causes of cellulite are:

1. Collagen degeneration
2. Reduced glycosaminoglycans
3. Congested liver

Cause 1: Collagen Degeneration

Cellulite results when subdermal fat cells push out through the columns of connective tissue. But why this process destroys connective tissue, and what causes the deterioration, is not clear or agreed upon by researchers. Some maintain that collagen is weakened by nutritional deficiencies; others think it is caused by hormonal imbalances, others by toxic build up, and still others believe impaired cardiovascular circulation is the culprit.

The disagreement over possible causes is probably due to the fact that one cause is not generally found without another. We often experience toxic over-load, dehydration, and nutritional deficiencies at the same time. Additionally, deficiencies lead to toxicity due to our organs' impaired ability to eliminate toxins. It might not be easy to find a group of test subjects who don't have nutritional deficiencies, hormonal imbalances, and a toxic liver all at the same time.

You know that weak collagen might be your problem if:

- Your diet mostly consists of prepared foods.
- You are anorexic or bulimic.
- You have wrinkles and sagging skin.
- You are a vegetarian and don't eat adequate or complete protein.
- Most of your protein comes from overcooked meat.
- You don't eat much Vitamin C, zinc, or magnesium.
- You've had fluoride treatments at the dentist, drink fluoridated water, and use fluoride toothpaste. Fluoride reduces circulatory levels of a compound called glycosaminoglycan, which attracts water and hydrates our cells.

Lack of Collagen Building Nutrients

As we learned in the last chapter, there are many nutrients such as protein, Vitamin C, and zinc that are critical for the health of our connective tissue. If we don't eat enough quality protein and don't give our bodies the nutrients they need to synthesize that protein, our cells won't have the amino acid building blocks needed to regenerate collagen. This results in a weak supportive structure for our subcutaneous fat cells. Additionally, we need to supply our connective tissue with the actual compounds found in connective tissue. Bone broth, made by boiling the bones and joints of animals, contains these compounds. In the past (and in many parts of the world today), people avoided cellulite by using the whole animal and drinking the nutritious broth from their bones.

Cellular Dehydration

Dr. Howard Murad was instrumental in developing the "water principle" of cellulite. According to this theory, when our bodies don't have the nutrients they need, cells become damaged and less able to hold onto the water they need to be vibrant and healthy. Dehydrated cells do not function optimally and cannot repair and hydrate the skin. At this point, blood vessels, which are primarily composed of connective tissue, break down as well, further contributing to the problem by impeding their ability to transport water and nutrients to the skin.

Damaged blood vessels leak water and do not carry water through the body efficiently. This free-floating water, as Dr. Murad calls it, does our cells little good. The water is needed *inside* our cells, not floating around outside them. When a body is thirsty on a cellular level, the skin will appear dry, may form stretch marks and cellulite, and the skin may sag and wrinkle. To stay hydrated on a cellular level, we must give our bodies the nutrients they need to build the strong connective tissue and blood vessels needed to carry the water essential to our skin.

It's easy to understand how wrinkles are caused by dehydration—wrinkles actually look like dehydrated skin— but cellulite has the same root cause. The dermis becomes weaker and thinner as a result of the lack of water, giving room for fat cells to rise up into the dermis. The dried-out connective tissues shrink up as a result and essentially clamp down on the fat, causing the lumpy texture of cellulite. When connective tissues become severely dry and hard, they actually wrap around clumps of fat cells. This advanced cellulite will look particularly severe and can be painful.

Cellular dehydration can happen regardless of how much water a person drinks. The problem is not that the body isn't given enough water, but that the damage to circulatory tissues causes water to escape out of the cells. What is needed are nutrients to repair cell walls and connective tissue so that water can successfully travel to the affected site, thicken up the dermis, and essentially let go of the clumps of fat.

Cause 2: Glycosaminoglycans (GAGs)

The cells within our connective tissue are surrounded by what is called the extracellular matrix—a network of proteins and polysaccharides. Part of that matrix is made up of polysaccharide chains called glycosaminoglycans (GAGs), and the other part is made up of fibrous proteins, which include collagen and elastin. The GAGs attract massive amounts of water and are responsible for keeping our tissues hydrated. Hydration is imperative in maintaining the strength of connective tissues.

GAGs are synthesized primarily from glucosamine. The body can produce glucosamine out of glucose, but to reverse connective tissue damage you will probably need to take a glucosamine supplement, or, better yet, drink bone broth. The body is only equipped to make so much glucosamine, so any extra will need to come from your diet.

Effects of Fluoride on Glycosaminoglycans

There are many foods that cause connective tissue degradation. Sugar and vegetable oils are a couple of well-known culprits because they compromise the integrity of our cells. But there are chemicals practically forced upon us that also interfere with collagen formation. We don't know precisely how these chemicals impact us on a cellular level, but some of the more heavily researched, like fluoride, are now known to cause side effects.

Fluoride has long been used to prevent cavities and strengthen teeth, and there may be some short-term benefits. But some of the side effects are long-term. Research has shown that fluoride reduces circulatory levels of glycosaminoglycans (GAGs) by almost 30 percent. GAGs are very important for the health of our connective tissue. Hyaluronic acid, for example, can retain one thousand times its weight in water. This is very useful in plumping up our connective tissue and helping them maintain resiliency.

Our bodies make hyaluronic acid and other GAGs from glucosamine, which have traditionally been consumed in broths from bones. Not only do our modern diets not offer these important connective tissue building compounds, but the chemicals in our water and hygiene products further reduce their circulatory level. Reduced glycosaminoglycan levels can be responsible for dramatic changes in our connective tissue, so take caution before ingesting fluoride.

Hormones

As I mentioned in chapter 7, glucocorticoids impair the skin's ability to repair collagen. When glucocorticoids are high, fibroblasts are unable to produce new collagen. We know that glucocorticoids increase during pregnancy. This might be why previously cellulite-free women start to see it when they're pregnant.

Excess estrogen is another possible agent in weakening connective tissue. Estrogen dominance is a common hormonal imbalance. It is also responsible for the symptoms of PMS and other menstrual problems. Balancing estrogen—i.e., increasing progesterone—can do wonders for the look of the skin.

Several double-blind studies have been done to confirm this. In one, published in 2005 in the *British Journal of Dermatology*, Dr. Gregor Holzer and colleagues reported that topical progesterone cream increases skin firmness and elasticity. In addition to the studies performed with progesterone creams, there is quite a bit of anecdotal evidence supporting the role of progesterone in skin health. Menopausal women, many of whom experience a near 100 percent drop in progesterone, experience a significant increase in wrinkles and dry, itchy skin. When they start taking progesterone creams for hot flashes and other symptoms of menopause, not only do they start sleeping through the night, their skin complaints miraculously improve. This is because during episodes of hormonal imbalance, collagen suffers and the skin loses its elasticity.

Cause 3: Congested Lymph and Toxic Liver

Many researchers contend that there's more to cellulite than weakened collagen. If our detoxification systems—like the lymph and liver—are impaired, fat cells can become bloated with toxins. This can cause everything from headaches and allergies to cellulite.

The Lymphatic System

Welcome to our body's underground sewage system. This is where all the dirty runoff goes, keeping everything 'above' clean and functional. Much like a city, our bodies produce a lot of waste. Old cells die off and bacteria, viruses, and toxins need to be disposed of. With no cleanup system, we would start to look and feel pretty icky.

The lymphatic system tends to get outshined by the cardiovascular system, which *brings* nutrients to our cells via the blood. But the lymphatic system is just as important. As nutrients are delivered to our cells, metabolic waste is produced and must be carried away. Like the cardiovascular system, the lymphatic system is an extensive circulatory system of vessels that connect to nearly every cell in the body. Through those vessels flows lymph, a milky white fluid that carries waste out of the body. However, while the heart pumps our blood, it's our muscles that pump lymph. This is why exercise is critical for keeping our bodies clean and waste free.

Some researchers are convinced that cellulite arises when our lymphatic system gets congested, meaning that lymph is not flowing as it should, allowing waste to build up in our cells. This can happen when we live in a very polluted city, eat a highly toxic diet, produce an excess of toxins due to allergies, work at a stressful job, or avoid exercise.

You may have a congested lymphatic system if you:

- Have regularly or occasionally taken over the counter medication for things like headaches and injuries
- Have taken street drugs like marijuana or others
- Have been an excessive drinker at any time in your life or a regular drinker all of your life
- Smoke
- Live in a big, polluted city
- Generally wear synthetic clothing, cook with synthetic pots and pans, eat out of plastics
- Come into contact with plastics or other chemicals on a regular basis
- Eat fast food or packed food
- Don't exercise

Even if only one of these markers was an overwhelming yes, your liver may have become overburdened and, as a result, your lymphatic system may be overworked. When toxins and waste materials are not removed from our cells, they become inflamed and produce the bulge of cellulite.

Toxic Liver

Here's another theory: Ann Louise Gittleman, author of *The Fat Flush Plan*, believes that cellulite is caused by a toxic liver. She contends that flushing the liver and restoring its ability to filter toxins will eliminate cellulite.

> *"If either the incoming fresh blood, or the outgoing 'used' blood is restricted, free radicals start to build up and oxygen becomes scarce. This causes more damage to the circulation and impairs the function of the cells that manage the structure of the connective tissue. These cells are known as fibroblasts and when they malfunction, they cause two problems: They weaken the fibers that hold the fat cells in place, and they coat clumps of fat cells with impenetrable protein layers that prevent the circulation from reaching these areas."*

Strategies to Reduce Cellulite

There are hundreds of anti-cellulite plans available online and in books. They all come at the problem from different angles and each offers some valid information. But most of them miss the connection to collagen and hormonal balance. I doubt you will have much success eliminating cellulite by focusing on just exercise or just dry brushing or even just liver cleansing (I tried them all myself years ago). The best approach is to incorporate all of these recommendations into a whole body treatment plan. Not only will your thighs thank you, but your overall health will improve and, consequently, so will your quality of life.

The whole body approach to eliminating cellulite includes:

- Exercise
- Detox
- Nutrient-dense diet
- Antioxidants
- Elimination of processed foods
- Elimination of overcooked meats
- Hormone supplementation

- Weight loss
- Dry skin brushing and creams

Exercise

Exercise can help reduce and prevent cellulite by improving the circulation of lymph and blood alike, which removes toxins and delivers nutrients. It also helps to keep our hormones balanced, which is important for healthy connective tissue. However, exercise is not a one-stop cure. No matter what you've heard, walking every day will not do the trick. Exercise is just one part of your healthy lifestyle approach.

Another myth is that doing targeted exercises like leg lifts and butt exercises will reduce cellulite. I don't want to discourage you from any kind of strengthening routine, but spot reduction techniques alone will not diminish the appearance of cellulite (nor, I might add, will they reduce fat or spider veins in certain areas.)

Detox

Toxins can accumulate in fat cells and cause the cells to behave less than optimally. They can cause inflammation, leading to swelling of the fat cells. Toxins also reduce circulation, which will lead to fewer nutrients being available to the cells, and consequently weakened connective tissue.

Detoxification is not recommended while pregnant, however, because some of the toxins stored in our fat cells can be flushed into our blood stream. These toxins might then come in contact with the fetus. Any rigorous detoxification program should be postponed until pregnancy and breastfeeding have ended. Of course, common sense dictates that a pregnant or nursing mother should try to avoid coming into contact with new toxins.

Nutrient-Dense Diet

To repair and maintain healthy connective tissue we need good nutrition. There are many specific nutrients that you can eat and take as supplements which will help build a strong dermis layer. When a body has the right nutrients, the collagen network will thicken and fat cells will be hidden by the thicker dermis and epidermis. Chapter 12 offers a connective tissue-repair diet.

Antioxidants

One of the most ubiquitous forms of toxins are *free radicals*. Free radicals are molecules that lack an electron. All molecules must have an even number of electrons. When they lose one, they are called free radicals. Free radicals are found in certain foods and created in our bodies.

External sources of free radicals:

- Cigarette smoke
- Alcohol
- Processed foods
- Old food
- Overcooked or burnt food
- Preservatives
- Chlorine
- Pesticides
- Herbicides
- Household cleaners, fingernail polish, paints, glues, new carpet
- Exhaust fumes
- Pollution
- Too much sun

Internal sources of free radicals:

- Bacterial and viral infections
- Allergic reactions to pollen, dander, and foods
- Lack of sleep
- Emotional stress
- Physical stress in the form of injuries or high-intensity exercise
- Partially digested foods from eating too quickly or insufficient enzymes
- Overeating
- Constipation
- Hormone imbalances

A free radical is a wild molecule. In its quest to pick up a new electron, it not only destroys everything it bumps into, it turns other molecules into free radicals. This free radical attack—called oxidative stress—can only be calmed by eating natural antioxidants.

Anti-oxidant Super Foods	
Green tea	Fresh, raw carrot juice
Red wine	Cherries, goji berries, and other berries
Dark chocolate	Sweet potatoes
Pomegranates	Spinach

Eliminate Processed Foods

Foods that contribute to cellulite are those that contain toxins or disrupt hormone balance. The Standard American Diet is the perfect recipe for cellulite because it is toxic, inflammatory, high glycemic, and deficient. All of these elements contribute both to weakening of cells and connective tissue and to the congestion of lymph.

Eliminate Overcooked Protein

Some researchers believe that the overconsumption of protein is partly at fault for the prevalence of cellulite. I agree with this claim to some degree. Much of the protein foods that Americans consume today are overcooked. Overcooking meats creates toxins and destroys amino acids, the building blocks the body needs to generate new collagen.

Natural Hormone Supplementation

While you will be able to bring your body back into balance by changing your diet and adopting a healthier lifestyle, you can help speed the balancing process by using a natural progesterone cream. Reducing the progesterone to estrogen ratio is often very helpful in improving skin conditions since excess estrogen is often responsible for the fibroblast's inability to generate new collagen tissue.

Human Growth Hormone (HGH) is another supplementation women have found useful. According to Dr. Marcelle Pick, OB/GYN of Women to Women, HGH rejuvenates skin. We release human growth hormone when we fast and in even greater amounts when we exercise while fasting.

Weight Loss

Losing weight can help take some pressure off of the subdermal fat layer, making cellulite less apparent. But chances are, if you do nothing else to combat it, you will still have the problem. And without a doubt, if weight loss is your only strategy, you will not pass the squeeze test. The proof of your weakened connective tissue will still be apparent when you cross your legs or press into your skin.

Dry Skin Brushing

Dry skin brushing with a loofah or a dry bristle brush encourages circulation and can help detoxify the lymph. By applying the proper dry brushing technique, a person can promote lymphatic drainage and improve circulation to the cells.

Cellulite Creams

Products for cellulite usually contain natural extracts, including caffeine, essential oils like horse chestnut, and other herbal extracts. The expectation is that these extracts will penetrate the dermis layer of the skin and deliver the nutrients to the connective tissue. For the most part, this is not possible because the dermis layer is protected by the epidermis. The epidermis acts as a shield so that chemicals cannot penetrate the body. Hence, most of the cellulite creams on the market are worthless for cellulite reduction and are at best just decent moisturizers.

There are certain products, however, which contain subdermal carriers. Well-formulated products such as these are generally very expensive and results are short-lived. Delivering collagen to the dermis layer or reducing local inflammation can be effective temporarily, but, as we know, the problem comes from within.

Body Wraps

Topical agents like antioxidants and anti-inflammatories applied in a body wrap can effectively add nutrition deep into the skin. Wraps that include caffeine and other methylxanthines (diuretics and muscle relaxants) are effective in temporarily dehydrating the treated area. Procedures that utilize methylxanthines reduce the swelling caused by excess water, thereby minimizing the appearance of cellulite. Frequent repeat treatments would be necessary to maintain results because, again, the actual cause is not being addressed.

Other Cosmetic Procedures

There are other more expensive and invasive procedures that will yield temporary results. Dermal fillers involving injections of fat, collagen, or hyaluronic acid will improve skin texture, but the effects wear off in time. Other temporarily effective treatments include chemical peels, non-ablative lasers,

Extracorporeal Acoustic Wave Therapy, iontophoresis (which uses electrical currents to help feed mineral salts directly into the body) and Endermologie, an electrical subdermal massager.

My Success Eliminating Cellulite

I developed cellulite when I was very young because, as a vegetarian, I lived on processed vegetable oils, overcooked soy protein, and refined carbohydrates. I also drank a lot of coffee and engaged in other poor lifestyle habits. Surprisingly, when I eliminated these things, I did not see the problem resolve right away. When I learned about the Paleo diet and started eating the way our ancestors did, the cellulite disappeared. I didn't use any anti-cellulite treatments, creams, or herbs; I simply changed my diet. Over the years, I have discovered that I have to be careful. My connective tissue isn't so thick that I can eat whatever I want and still look beautiful. When I get lax with my diet and eat inflammatory or dehydrating foods, the cellulite becomes visible again.

CHAPTER 9

Varicose Veins and Hemorrhoids

Varicose veins are veins that have become enlarged and sinuous. They are usually located on the legs. When they are located in the rectal area they are called hemorrhoids. During pregnancy, they sometimes develop on the vulva as well. Due to the many changes that take place during pregnancy, all types of varicose veins are common during this time.

Anatomy of a Vein

In order to understand what makes a vein varicose, let's take a moment to understand what a vein is and how it functions in the body. While we often think of veins as the carriers of blood flow to and from the heart, veins actu-

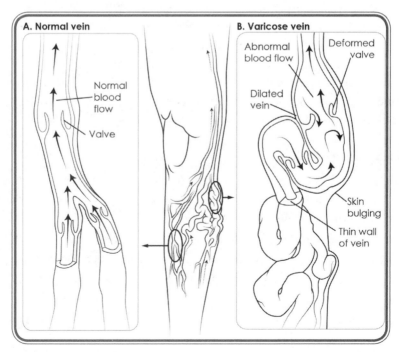

ally only work in on direction: They are the vessels which carry blood *back* to the heart. The arteries are the vessels that carry blood *away* from the heart.

In order for a vein to push blood up the legs and against gravity it must have a system of valves in place to prevent the flow of blood backwards. Our blood vessels are composed mostly of connective tissue, and so vein walls and valves are as vulnerable to deterioration as the skin.

As connective tissue weakens, so do the valves, allowing blood to flow backwards. This thins the lining of the vein, which in turn makes it swell and protrude through the skin. This is what we call varicose veins.

Risk Factors

Pregnancy

Many factors can increase a person's likelihood of developing varicose veins, but pregnancy is by far the greatest cause. During pregnancy, blood volume increases up to 50 percent, stressing the vessel walls and causing them to en-large. In the last trimester, the enlarged and heavy uterus puts pressure on the large vein of the right side, called the inferior vena cava. This can slow the return of blood from the lower extremities, which increases the pressure on the veins below the uterus, causing them to become even more swollen. Additionally, progesterone, which is significantly elevated during pregnancy, causes the vein walls to relax, allowing them to swell more easily. And as we have already learned, glucocorticoids can impair our ability to repair the connective tissue that makes up the walls of our vessels.

In addition to the above, hemorrhoids are common among pregnant women because elevated progesterone slows down the intestinal tract, con-tributing to constipation. Straining and pushing can cause hemorrhoids when vein walls are already weak.

Risk Factors Include:

* **Inactivity**—Veins, unlike arteries, do not rely on the pump of the heart to move the blood. Veins must utilize a collection of skeletal muscles to push the blood up to the heart.

* **Hormonal imbalance**—Puberty, pregnancy, menopause, and birth control pills are all risk factors in the formation of varicose veins be-cause they increase estrogen, thereby weakening connective tissue.

* **Obesity**—Excess weight can put significant pressure on the veins, im-peding blood flow. Additionally, muscles of obese people are weaker

than those of their thinner counterparts and do a poor job of pushing blood back up to the heart. This allows the blood to pool and varicose pockets to form.

+ **Age**—As we age, connective tissue throughout the body can weaken, rendering the valves insufficient and unable to do their job.

+ **Heredity**—Some people are born with weak vein valves, which can increase the risk. Researchers have observed that about half of all people who have varicose veins have a family member who has them too. But this doesn't tell us much since dietary and lifestyle habits also tend to run in families.

Symptoms of Varicose Veins and Hemorrhoids

Varicose veins may cause little to no discomfort, or they may cause the legs to feel heavy and achy. The skin around the veins may itch or throb or feel like it's burning. The symptoms tend to be worse at the end of the day and may contribute to fatigue.

Hemorrhoids and Vulvar Varicosities

Hemorrhoids can cause significant pain, particularly while straining during a bowel movement. They typically range in size from a pea to a grape and can be inside the rectum or protrude through the anus. They may be itchy and mildly uncomfortable or even excruciating. Sometimes they cause rectal bleeding, especially during a bowel movement. Symptoms tend to improve after giving birth and usually will totally clear up within a year of delivery.

Vulvar varicosities can also be quite uncomfortable or painful and, in some cases, can swell very large.

Spider Veins

Varicose veins sometimes feed increased pressure into the capillaries, causing spider veins. Spider veins are smaller, enlarged capillaries that usually, but not always, appear in a sunburst pattern. These visible veins do not cause any discomfort and usually clear up after delivery.

How to Relieve
the Pain of Hemorrhoids

If hemorrhoids have already developed and you're still pregnant, your main concern is to get relief. While strengthening vein walls is possible, it takes time; the body will have a hard time repairing the tissue while there is still significant pressure on the rectum and veins are enlarged.

+ **Apply ice**. When hemorrhoids become swollen and inflamed, ice will help reduce inflammation and relieve the pain. You can use an ice pack several times a day.

+ **Use a witch hazel cold compress**. Witch hazel is a natural, inexpensive anti-inflammatory distilled from the witch hazel plant. A cold compresses saturated with witch hazel cannot only reduce inflammation and pressure, it can also help prevent hemorrhoids.

+ **Keep the area clean**. Gently but thoroughly wipe after each bowel movement using soft, unscented, white toilet tissue, followed by an unscented, alcohol free baby wipe.

+ **Avoid constipation**. Constipation puts a lot of pressure on the veins of the rectum.

+ **Avoid excess fiber**. Conventional wisdom suggests increasing fiber to relive constipation, but this is not a good strategy for those suffering from hemorrhoids. Fiber is indigestible and can make bowel movements quite large, putting even greater pressure on the hemorrhoids, and causing pain.

Reversal and Prevention
of Varicose Veins and Hemorrhoids

Varicose veins and hemorrhoids often improve by themselves within three to four months after giving birth, though sometimes it takes longer. If the diet and lifestyle are not supportive, however, they may never be totally eliminated.

This is where good nutrition and fitness come in. Strong connective tissue and active muscles are the key to reversing and preventing varicose veins and hemorrhoids. When vein walls and valves are strong, they can withstand stretching. When a woman maintains her fitness, blood can flow through the vein as intended and not pool up in sections.

Pregnancy is a trying time for the body in many ways. Pregnant women must take extra care to pamper themselves. By this, I don't mean sitting in front of the TV all day with feet up and one hand in the chip bag. While that may sound like pampering to some, it is definitely not what the body needs. The body needs special foods and exercise to be strong and resilient.

To prevent varicosities a pregnant woman should:

- **Exercise daily and throughout the day**. Even a brisk walk around the block a few times a day can improve circulation, although, I would recommend more exercise than that for most pregnant women. The best exercises for strong, healthy blood flow are those which strengthen the muscles since these are in charge of pushing blood back up through the veins to the heart.

- **Keep weight down**. Staying within a healthy weight range for each stage of pregnancy will keep the pressure of excess body fat off of the veins and help keep the muscles stronger.

- **Do Kegel exercises**. Kegels increase circulation in the rectal area and help to keep blood moving through those veins. However, since Kegel exercises strengthen the muscles around the anus considerably, extra care should be taken not to strain while making a bowel movement. Straining puts significant pressure on the veins of the rectum, which can lead to hemorrhoids. For specific instructions on how to do Kegel exercises, see chapter 10.

- **Elevate the feet occasionally**. Whenever possible, elevating the legs will allow the blood to flow with gravity instead of against it. You can keep your feet elevated on a pillow while lying down.

- **Move often**. Don't sit or stand for long periods without taking breaks to move around. Remember that the muscles are responsible for sending the blood through the veins. Being inactive for too long impedes blood flow.

- **Sleep on the left side**. Since the inferior vena cava is on the right side, lying on the left side relieves the vein of the weight of the uterus, thus decreasing pressure on the veins temporarily. Wedging a pillow behind the back will keep you from rolling over on the right side.

- **Wear special support hose**. Compression stockings (available from medical supply stores and pharmacies) act by compressing the valves in the veins, making them more functional and lessening the venous reflux, or backward flow of blood, away from the heart. They're tight at the ankle and get looser as they go up the leg, which makes it easier for blood to flow back up toward your heart. They can help prevent swelling and may keep your varicose veins from getting worse. They only work while they are being worn and are notably effective in preventing already-developed varicose veins from getting worse.

There are also special vein-strengthening herbs. These are considered safe during pregnancy:

- **Butcher's Broom** contains the compound ruscogenins. These substances decrease inflammation while simultaneously constricting the vein. Butcher's Broom can be taken internally as a whole herb extract. A compress with the herb can also be applied externally.

- **Rosemary** is a common household herb that is very high in antioxidants and known to improve circulation to the veins. It can be used liberally in foods and applied as a compress.

- **Flavonoid** compounds are commonly found in many foods we eat every day, including onions, apple peels, and the white part of oranges. Flavonoids reduce fragility of the veins and help to tone muscles.

- **St. John's Wort** is commonly known to relieve depression, but it also reduces inflammation. The herb can be used internally (as capsules or tea) or externally. St. John's Wort loses its medicinal properties if air-dried, so use fresh or freeze-dried.

Treating Constipation

Constipation is the bane of pregnant women worldwide. This is partly due to the poor eating habits that many pregnant women adopt, like avoiding fresh and fermented foods or choosing a diet high in refined foods and sugar. But it's also a side effect of the changes in hormones (progesterone relaxes smooth muscle tissue, which is what controls bowel movements) and the movement of the bowels (when the uterus enlarges, it displaces the intestines and pushes them up against the stomach and back wall) that happen to every pregnant woman.

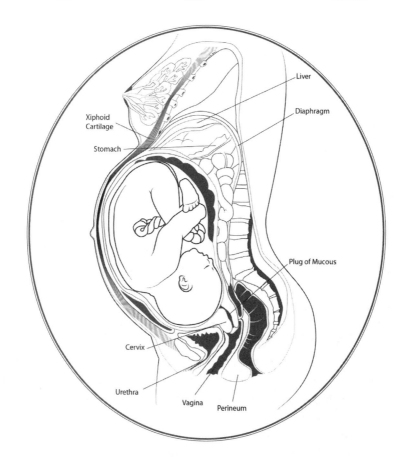

Peristalsis

The motility of our stool, or bowel movements, is entirely dependent upon the nearly constant pushing and contracting of our intestinal smooth muscle—what is called peristalsis.

Smooth muscle is controlled unconsciously: We cannot tell ourselves when to poop, it just happens. The best way improve peristalsis is not with fiber, as conventional wisdom has led us to believe, but by improving gut flora, reducing inflammation, lowering stress, and improving nutrition.

Chief Causes of Constipation

- High fiber diet
- Heavily processed diets
- Nutritional deficiencies
- Low-fat diets

- Regular laxative use
- Conscious suppression
- Antibiotics
- Mercury fillings
- Drug use
- Alcohol abuse
- Stress
- Drinking too much water

A Word On Fiber

Americans have been told for years that they should eat a high fiber diet in order to push the stool out of the gut. While it often works well at first, fiber is essentially a laxative that, in time, can cause the bowel to become dependent, effectively reducing peristaltic sensitivity. Once that happens, the gut is full of bulky, impacted feces, and no amount of fiber will push it out.

Healthy bowel movements are not achieved simply by dropping something heavy into the intestines to push the stool out. It's not like an object being pulled by gravity through a vertical pipe. The small intestine, which digests and absorbs food, is about 20 feet long and looks a little like a roller-coaster track. The large intestine, which absorbs water from waste and creates the stool, is also called the colon and consists of four sections (ascending, transverse, descending, and stigmoid) that travel up, over, and down the other side of the small intestine, ending in the rectum. There is no pushing. There is only peristalsis, our own body's reflexes.

I was constipated while I was pregnant the first time and so I went with conventional wisdom and added fiber to my diet. I gradually added more and more, until I was up to about 40 grams of fiber, all from vegetable sources. At no point along the way did my bowels improve. In fact, I became bloated, had stomachaches, and developed hemorrhoids due to straining. It was very uncomfortable. It wasn't until years later, when I started looking into the cause of constipation and discovered the book *Fiber Menace,* by Konstantin Monastyrsky, that I realized fiber was not some magic solution to constipation. This is not to say that some amount of fiber is not necessary. In fact, some amount of soluble fiber is beneficial for the microbes that populate our gut. But it needs to come from food sources and not as a fiber supplement. Fibrous vegetables also contain magnesium, which is necessary for bowel movements.

Conscious Suppression of Peristalsis

Constant conscious suppression of the urge to defecate—because we're in a hurry, stuck in traffic, at a concert, or in a conversation—can cause constipation over time. Doing this repeatedly sends the signal to, in effect, silence the scream we don't intend to listen to. Suppression is a valuable mechanism: It could be fatal to run to the bathroom in the middle of an earthquake, for example. It's just not something to get into the habit of doing on a regular basis.

Tips On Avoiding Constipation:

- **Repair gut flora**. Restoring healthy gut flora is critical to resolving constipation. But since constipation itself is damaging to a healthy bacterial population, the gut flora needs to be repaired before constipation can be reversed. Sounds like a Catch-22, right? Fortunately, there are ways to get the bowels moving even before the situation is resolved. Start with a magnesium glycinate supplement, then, once the bowels are moving, include fermented foods and drinks to boost healthy gut flora.

- **Eat anti-inflammatory foods**. A big contributor to constipation is inflammation. You can reduce inflammation by avoiding drugs, alcohol, medications, processed foods, and overcooked meats. Taking cod liver oil and eating anti-inflammatory foods (fish, eggs, dark chocolate, etc.) will lower inflammation.

- **Eat some foods raw**. They generally contain more nutrients and enzymes than their cooked counterparts. They also contain more water and do not contain damaged fats or denatured proteins, both of which can contribute to inflammation.

- **Favor soluble fiber over insoluble**. Insoluble fiber can be irritating to the gut while soluble fiber offers food for good bacteria. Foods with soluble fiber include bananas, potatoes, mushrooms, apples, and many others.

- **Eat animal fat**. Low fat diets contribute to constipation. Fat stimulates the release of the bile that stimulates peristalsis. If a person does not eat fat and bile is not released, then the whole digestive process stalls. Eating too much fat, on the other hand—i.e., more fat than you can manage to digest in one sitting—will cause the fat to seep, undigested, into the intestines, bringing water into the bowels and possibly causing diarrhea. How much fat is too much fat depends on the person and how much bile the individual produces.

- **Manage stress**. Stress brings peristalsis to a halt. Americans today rarely have a need for flight or fight (which induces peristalsis suppression). What they do have is all sorts of stresses which prevent us from going to the bathroom. Do everything you can to relax. This may mean doing yoga, winding down at the end of the day, or adding half an hour in the morning so that you have time for a bowel movement rather than just rushing out the door.

- **Avoid fermentable carbohydrates (FODMAPs)**. Lactose, fructose, and other carbohydrates are not easily digested by many people. When these pass through the digestive system, undigested, they cause inflammation and irritation to the intestinal lining. Many foods fall under the FODMAPs label but some of the more common ones include: apples, mango, pear, peas, asparagus, cabbage, garlic, onions, avocado, and mushrooms. If you have suspected that some of these foods cause digestive troubles, you may want to read further about FODMAPs sensitivity.

- **Check your stomach acid levels**. Stomach acid is often low in people with gut issues. If you have trouble digesting meat or if you have low B12, despite the fact that you do eat meat, you probably have low stomach acid. You can do a test with some inexpensive betain HCL supplements to determine your stomach acid levels. Eat a meal containing about six ounces of meat. About midway through your meal, take one pill. If within a few hours you feel a burning sensation in your chest, your stomach acid is sufficient. If you don't feel a burning sensation, try the test at your next meal with two pills. Perform the test, increasing your dosage, until you feel the burning sensation. The more pills you must take, the lower your stomach acid. Consult your nutritionist or naturopathic doctor for guidance if you determine your stomach acid is low. Taking HCL with high protein meals will improve your digestion.

- **Try switching or eliminating your iron supplement**. Iron supplements can cause constipation. Switching to a different form of iron can resolve the issue; better yet, get iron from nutritious foods like red meat and dark, leafy greens.

- **Drink water**. But not too much! Excess water can cause constipation as much as too little can. The basic recommendation is to drink 6-8 glasses of water per day. But much of the water we need comes from the food we eat and other drinks like tea, milk, and juice. If you are mostly avoiding processed foods, then your actual water requirement should be more like 2-3 glasses per day.

- **Add magnesium**. Magnesium is required for the movement of smooth muscle. Without adequate amounts, our bowels will stop. Magnesium glycinate, which is a chelated form of magnesium, does not cause bowel dependence. Foods high in magnesium include halibut, bananas, spinach, artichokes, nuts, and dark chocolate.

- **Avoid dairy**. Raw dairy can be very healing for some, but for others who do not tolerate lactose, casein, or other milk proteins, dairy can create inflammation. If this is true for you, try substituting ghee, which has no casein or lactose, for butter.

- **Avoid caffeine and coffee**. While coffee does act as a diuretic, what we are trying to achieve is a return to natural peristalsis, not forced peristalsis. Additionally, caffeine is dehydrating and can rob the bowels of necessary water. It also causes the release of cortisol, the stress hormone, which suppresses peristalsis. It should be avoided by anyone with digestive problems and by pregnant women in general.

- **Don't smoke**. If you're pregnant or breastfeeding, you probably don't smoke anyway, but I had to throw it in there. Cigarette smoke kills off healthy bacteria, reduces circulation, and causes inflammation.

- **Stop taking prescription medication if possible**. Constipation is one of the many side effects of prescription meds. Consider finding a natural healing alternative.

- **Exercise every day**. Regular exercise increases circulation, improves muscle tone, and reduces inflammation.

- **Squat**. Toilets put us in a very unnatural position for elimination. If you've ever pooped out in the woods you know that you don't do it sitting on a chair, you do it in a squatting position. Squatting encourages elimination by putting gentle pressure on the bowels. Chairs have basically replaced the squat in our culture and now Americans rarely assume that position (unlike many Asians who spend hours in it). Try to squat occasionally throughout the day to improve digestion. In a true squatting position you should feel the knees against your chest. The elbows should not rest on the knees. Or consider purchasing a Squatty Potty (www.squattypotty.com), a sort of stool that you can place in front of the toilet.

- **Treat hemorrhoids**. If hemorrhoids are large and obstructing bowel movement, steps should be taken to reduce inflammation. Note that fiber can actually make stools larger, leading to more pain.

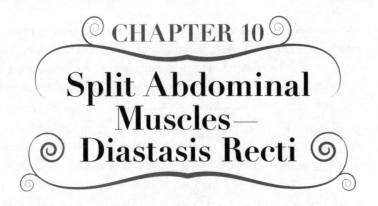

CHAPTER 10

Split Abdominal Muscles— Diastasis Recti

It's bad enough that you lose your small waist after pregnancy, but there are functionality issues with the changes of a postpartum abdomen as well, like incontinence and lower back pain. Thankfully, with a little dedication to strengthening the abdominals and connective tissue, your abdomen can both look and feel like nothing happened (or close enough!).

Physiology of the Abdomen

The abdominal muscles consist of the rectus abdominis (also known as the "abs") and the three sheets of muscle that form a sheath around it: the external obliques, the internal obliques, and the transverse abdominis.

The rectus abdominis runs down the front on either side of the midline. It originates at the pubis and ends in the cartilage of the fifth, sixth, and seventh ribs. Running across the rectus abdominis are three creases of tendons that give the abdomen its washboard look. The rectus abdominis and obliques are important for bending sideways, for trunk rotation, and for stabilizing the trunk when getting up from lying down. They are also used for pushing out babies and feces (though they probably shouldn't be).

The transverse abdominis does not aid in the movement of the body but plays an important role in the forceful expiration of air from the lungs. It also helps to stabilize the back and organs.

Separation of the Rectus Abdominis

The rectus abdominis is actually two parallel muscles fused at the midline by connective tissue called the linea alba. Under certain conditions these muscles can become separated or stretched as the integrity of the linea alba is compromised. This is especially common during pregnancy, but it can also occur in anyone who habitually puts pressure on the rectus abdominis because of weakened connective tissue.

The hormonal changes that take place during pregnancy soften connective tissue, allowing them to stretch. As the uterus grows near the end of pregnancy, pressure is exerted on the linea alba. As the connective tissue weakens, the linea alba can become so thin and stretched that the rectus abdominis muscles appear further apart. (In advanced cases, the connective tissue can actually begin to tear, leading to hernias that must be treated with surgery.) This separation of the two sides of the rectus abdominis is called Diastasis recti abdominis, and it occurs in at least 50-60 percent of postpartum women.

How to Tell If You Have Diastasis Recti

If your belly is not fat and you are not bloated, yet it sticks out as if it were, diastasis recti might be the cause. While the following symptoms have a number of possible causes, they are common among those with diastasis recti:

- People think you are pregnant when you're not.
- You can see a gap running down the midline of your abdomen.
- You suffer from incontinence.
- You've had a Cesarean section.
- You have back problems.
- You have developed an outie belly button since childhood.

After the birth of your baby, if you notice that your belly has a triangular shape when getting up from lying on your back, you probably have some thinning of the linea alba. If you see a cone-shaped bulge in this midline area, your uterus or another organ may be pressing up against the thinned linea alba. If your diastasis recti is not this advanced and you're still not sure, you can do the finger width test.

Simple Test for Diastasis Recti

Lie down on your back with knees bent and feet planted on the floor. Place the tips of two fingers on the midline of the abdomen, one inch above the belly button. Do a small crunch upwards (gently round your head, neck and shoulders off the floor). If you feel a gap larger than two fingers between the muscles, you have diastasis recti. You can do the test in two additional places, at the belly button and below the belly button, to confirm.

Don't be surprised if the gap is greater than four fingers width. This is not uncommon. You probably won't suffer any serious health problems or be stuck with this for the rest of your life. Disastasis recti is repairable even in advanced stages. Ann Wendel of Prana Physical Therapy in Alexandria. VA, says that "it is never too late to treat a diastasis; it just requires time and commitment to heal it."

Before I tell you how to prevent and repair diastasis, let's take a moment to understand how the linea alba thins and separates.

Contributing Factors

Weak Abdominal Muscles

Keeping the muscles strong during and before pregnancy appears to be important in preventing this condition. Researchers in the study entitled *Incidence of Diastasis Recti Abdominis During the Childbearing Year* noted that :

> *"...women who, at the time of testing, fit the criteria as non-exercisers, but who had exercised vigorously before pregnancy or months before testing, still demonstrated well-toned, strong abdominal walls. Diastasis recti abdominis was absent in all of those women who had been conscientious exercisers before the onset of pregnancy."*

Forward Pressure on the Rectus Abdominis

Excessive exercising of the abdominal muscles with crunches or forward bending sit-ups puts pressure on the linea alba and, in time, can wear down the connective tissue. Crunches and sit-ups are not a good method for supporting abdominal integrity. Turning at the waist and other natural movements are always a better option, pregnant or otherwise.

Excess Weight Gain

Excess weight disrupts a woman's hormone balance, which can lead to a weakening of connective tissues in general. The additional pressure of significant belly fat further undermines the linea alba.

Cesarean Section

Women who have had a Cesarean section will usually show some signs of this condition since the abdominal muscles must be incised and pulled apart to remove the baby.

Potential Complications

Usually diastasis recti does not present serious complications. However, it does affect quality of life, contributing to:

+ **Cone-shaped or bulging abdomen**—Instead of having a flat sheet of muscle, you have two sides of muscles pointing upwards and towards each other and not quite meeting in the middle. This makes the belly appear cone-shaped, especially when you get up from lying on your back.

+ **Chronic lower back pain**—This is common in people with weak abdominal muscles in general.

+ **Hunched posture**—The abdominal muscles help to keep the back straight. When they are weak, posture suffers.

+ **Digestive troubles**—Bad posture can affect digestion.

+ **Difficulty lifting**—Toned abdominal muscles are required for lifting heavy objects.

+ **Inactivity**—Abdominal muscles are required for all sorts of mundane movements, such as turning, pulling, and getting up. Weak abdominal muscles can lead to a vicious cycle of inactivity and injuries.

+ **Umbilical hernia**—If the linea alba actually tears, which sometimes happens along the line of a previous incision, a gap can form between the muscles, causing the uterus or other organs to bulge through. This is something you would notice in the third trimester or after delivery.

+ **Incontinence**—Weak pelvic floor muscles can lead to incontinence.

How to Prevent and Repair Diastasis Recti

Prevention and repair of diastasis recti involves a balance of gentle, effective exercise and a nutrient-dense diet that supports the regrowth of connective tissue. Here are the four key ways to avoid and prevent the condition:

1. Keep weight down
2. Avoid forward forceful movements, such as sit-ups and getting straight up from lying down on your back
3. Maintain or rebuild abdominal muscle tone
4. Eat sufficient protein, minerals, and vitamins to support tissue repair as the linea alba stretches during pregnancy

The best workouts for the abdominals involve balance and natural turning movements, which is why yoga is an ideal option for pregnant women. Many yoga centers have pre-natal classes and, if not, there are pre-natal adjustments that you can do on your own. Swimming is also great for full body muscle strengthening, including the abs. The exercises to avoid are crunches, sit-ups, and heavy lifting. These put undue pressure on the abdominals, increasing susceptibility to the condition. The same principles for preventing the condition should be followed for repair, but instead of maintaining muscle tone we will seek to rebuild it.

Ann Wendel, PT, ATC, CMTPT of Prana Physical Therapy in Alexandria, Virginia, provided the following exercises and descriptions to help pregnant and postpartum women rebuild abdominal muscles and repair diastasis recti. One very important note: Pregnant women *must not* perform exercises while lying on their backs after the first trimester.

Alignment Exercises

Before beginning any of the following stabilization exercises, you'll want to find and maintain proper alignment. Improper alignment can cause lower back, shoulder, and neck pain, as well as other complications (see chapter 13).

Quadriped Alignment
Start in a tabletop position, on your hands and knees, with hands flat on the floor, wrists directly below your shoulders, and knees directly below your

hips. Look at the floor but keep your neck and head neutral (not hanging or raised) by imagining a line running from your tailbone, up your spine, and out through the top of your head. Lengthen your body along that line.

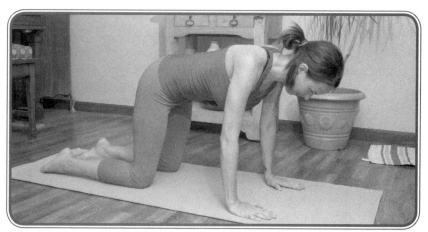

Figure 1: Quadriped alignment

Now have someone place a rod or foam roller along your spine, as shown in Figure 2. You should have three points of contact with the foam roller: the back of your head, the area between your shoulder blades, and your tailbone. If you notice that the foam roller is not connecting with any of those points, adjust your position until you feel all three.

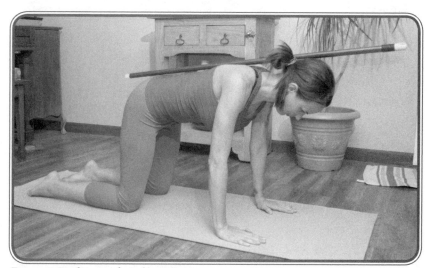

Figure 2: Finding perfect alignment

Progression 1: While keeping the three points of contact, practice doing a Kegel exercise: Take a breath in, and as you exhale, gently lift the pelvic floor up along the imaginary line that runs up your spine and through the top of your head). Repeat the progression a few times until it feels natural to you.

Progression 2: Once you have mastered progression 1, allow your belly to totally relax and hang down while still keeping your three points of contact with the foam roller; be careful not to allow your back to arch. Do your Kegel exercise, and this time lift your belly button toward your spine without rounding through your back. The key here is to keep the tailbone in contact with the foam roller. Relax and repeat several times.

Progression 3: Perform another Kegel, lifting the belly button toward the spine while maintaining your three points of contact. Now, take a deep breath in and out *without* releasing the belly button from the spine. Keep practicing until you can do several complete breaths in a row, relaxing in between as needed.

Awareness of Anterior Pelvic Tilt (Arch)

Anterior pelvic tilt—when the front of the pelvis drops and the back rises up—is due to months of carrying the weight of a baby on the front of your body and is common among postpartum women. It's the excessive curve in the lower back (see Figure 3) that you see when you stand or lie down. What we want instead is to keep the lumbar spine and pelvis in a more neutral position.

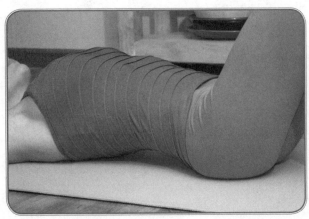

Figure 3: Anterior pelvic tilt (arch)

Finding a Neutral Spine

To encourage a neutral spine, lie on your back with knees bent. Draw your belly button slightly up and slightly in so that your pelvis is tilted and your lower back comes into contact with the floor. Think of it as drawing your belly away from the zipper on a pair of tight pants. Hold this position while you breathe in and out. Repeat 10 times.

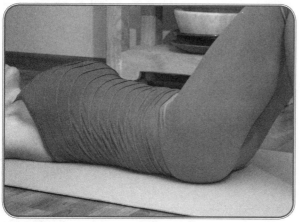

Figure 4: Neutral spine

Exercises for Pregnancy and Postpartum

Scapular Stabilization Starting Position: "Sinking"

Assume the tabletop position on your hands and knees. Allow the area between your shoulder blades to sink toward the floor. Keep your elbows straight the entire time.

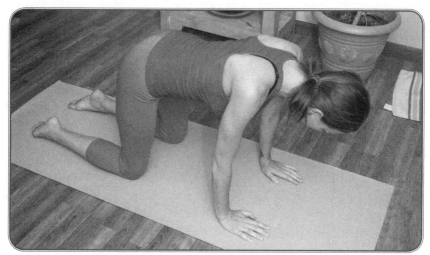

Figure 5: Scapular stabilization, start position

Scapular Stabilization End Position: "Push Up Plus"

From the "sinking" position, inhale then exhale slowly as you push through your hands and arms, lifting the area between your shoulder blades toward the ceiling. Hold for 2 seconds, then relax. Repeat 10 times.

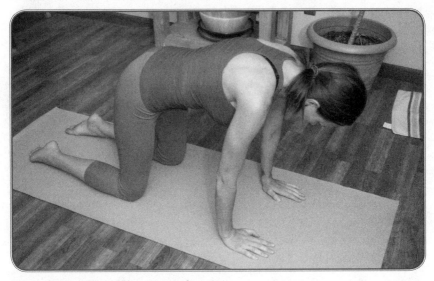

Figure 6: Scapular stabilization, end position

Side-Lying Clamshell: Starting Position

Lie on your right side with your hips "stacked" and in line with your spine. Your knees will be bent. Extend your right arm under your head and stabilize with your left hand on the floor in front of you.

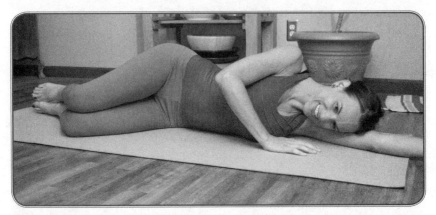

Figure 7: Side-lying clamshell, position 1

Side-Lying Clamshell: Position 2

Keeping your belly scooped toward your spine and ribs knitted together (see Knitting the Ribs Together in Postpartum Exercises, below), keep your feet touching and lift your left knee up toward the ceiling in a "clamshell." Check your form: Do not allow the hips to roll back during this movement; if it helps, imagine that there is a wall behind your back. You should feel the muscle on the side of your hip working as you do this movement. Hold the clamshell for 1-2 seconds, then lower the knee and relax. Perform 10 times on each side, inhaling when you relax and exhaling as you lift.

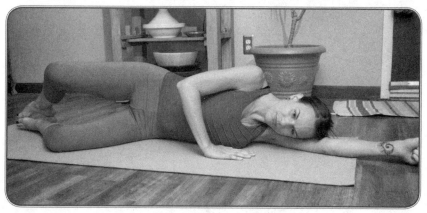

Figure 8: Side-lying clamshell, position 2

Squat with Pelvic Floor Integration

It is very important to work on proper static and dynamic posture during and after pregnancy. Simply put, this means that your ribs need to stay over your pelvis, so that your diaphragm and pelvic floor can work together. Keeping proper posture is difficult during the later stages of pregnancy, which makes it even more important to correct it in the early postpartum period.

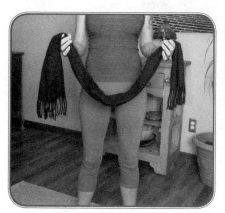

Step 1: Stand with feet wider than hip width apart, and feet slightly angled out. Your arms can be at your sides. The u-shaped band is illustrating that your pelvic floor should be relaxed in the starting position.

Figure 9:
Squat, step 1

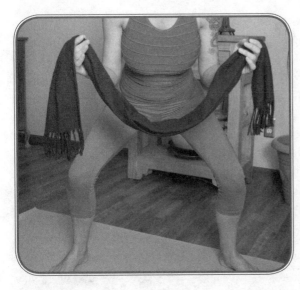

Figure 10:
Squat, step 2

Step 2: Inhale as you squat down as far as you comfortably can, keeping your pelvic floor relaxed (band is still relaxed) and your belly soft.

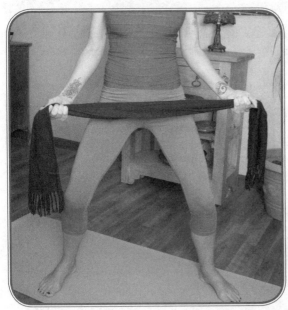

Figure 11:
Squat, step 3

Step 3: Exhale as you rise out of the squat, lifting the pelvic floor and using the deep abdominals to help push all the air out of your lungs. Taking the slack out of the band illustrates that the pelvic floor is drawn in and up, tightening the muscles. Repeat 10 times.

Postpartum Exercises

Knitting the Ribs Together

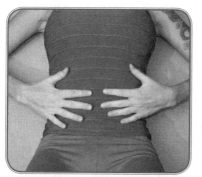

Figure 12: Knitting the ribs, step 1

Step 1: Now that you know how to achieve a neutral spine, you may work on bringing the ribs together. During pregnancy the abdominals are often overstretched, especially in the case of diastasis recti. You may even notice that your ribcage is wider than it used to be. Lie on the floor with a neutral spine and place your hands on top of your ribs. Feel how far apart the ribs are.

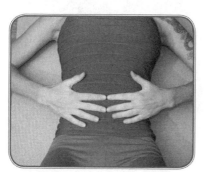

Figure 13: Knitting the ribs, step 2

Step 2: Now, imagine that you are lacing up a corset and bring the ribs closer together. Keep your neck relaxed as you find the muscles that bring the ribs together, using your hands for feedback.

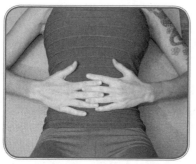

Figure 14: Knitting the ribs, step 3

Step 3: Once you get the ribs a bit closer together, keep them there as you hold the neutral spine position. Breathe one full breath in and out. Focus on breathing into your lower, back ribs.

Supine Marching

Assume the step 3 position of the rib-knitting exercise (belly toward spine, ribs knitted together). Bend your legs, feet on the floor, and lift one foot, pause for a second or two, then lower to floor. Alternate left and right feet for 10 repetitions. Breathe out as you raise each foot, breathe in as you return it to the floor. Make sure that your abdominals stay "scooped" and do not "pooch." Do not allow your lower back to lift off the floor at any point during the exercise.

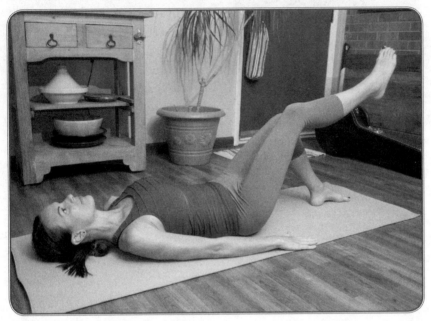

Figure 15: Supine marching

Knee Fold

Once you can perform 10 repetitions of Supine Marching without losing your form, progress to the Knee Fold exercise. Keep the Supine March position, but now lift your left foot off the ground and bring it to a supine tabletop. Keep your lower back on the floor and left leg in tabletop, then lift the right foot off the floor and align with the left. Lower your left foot to the floor, and then your right. Repeat this sequence: left leg up, right leg up, left leg down, right leg down. The trick is to really use your deep abdominals to keep your lower back and hips stabilized as you do the exercise. Perform 10 reps. Concentrate on breathing with the movements; do not hold your breath.

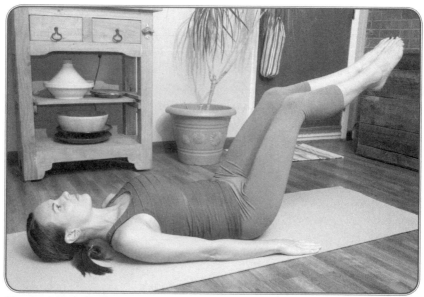

Figure 16: Knee Fold

Prone Swimming

This exercise is for stabilizing your spinal muscles. Lay on your stomach with your arms and legs extended. Lift your belly away from the floor by sucking your bellybutton into your spine. First lift your left arm and right leg an inch or two off the floor, reaching as long as possible. Keep your hips and spine from moving and your back from arching. Pause and hold for 1-2 seconds, then lower. Switch to the right arm and the left leg. Repeat 10 times, breathing in as you lower and out as you raise the opposing arm and leg.

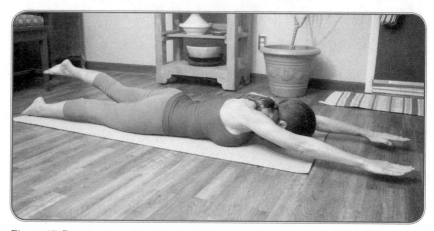

Figure 17: Prone swimming

Single Leg Glute Bridge

Start on your back with knees bent. Keep the spine in a neutral position and, pushing through your left foot, lift your hips and your right leg off the ground with the knee bent to about 90 degrees; keep your shoulders and upper back pressed into the floor. Squeeze your gluteal muscles (buttocks) to get as much hip extension as you can, while keeping your spine neutral; do not arch your lower back to get it higher. The focus here is on extending through the hip by squeezing the buttocks. Maintain a level pelvis—as in, don't let the hips tilt to the right or left.

If this exercise causes any back pain, or if you are unable to stabilize with the leg lifted, begin by performing the exercise with both feet on the floor, then progress to as you are able.

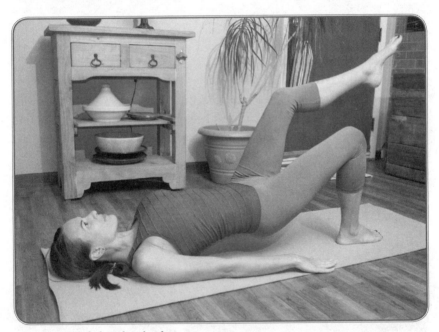

Figure 18: Single leg glute bridge

Repair for Extreme Cases

Splint

In extreme cases, if the abdominal muscles have thinned considerably, a splint may be required. That will bring the muscles close enough that they fuse back together.

> *"The splint should be specifically designed for treating rectus diastasis and must bring the rectus closer together, rather than just compressing the abdomen toward the spine," says physical therapist Ann Wendel. "It is important to wear the splint all the time, since we constantly utilize our abdominals in day to day activities, and going without the splint can put stress on the healing connective tissue and reopen the diastasis."*

Surgery

The cosmetic surgery procedure Abdominoplasty (more commonly known as a tummy tuck) is an option for women who don't want to exercise, who feel too much pain when exercising, who have a hernia, or who don't want to wear a splint. During the procedure, the fascia is tightened and the two sides of the abdomen are stitched together. Surgery isn't usually necessary, but it does allow for more rapid strengthening of the rectus abdominis.

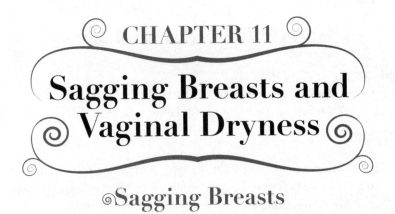

CHAPTER 11

Sagging Breasts and Vaginal Dryness

Sagging Breasts

We've already covered how collagen can prevent stretch marks, wrinkles, and cellulite, strengthen the joints, and keep your waist small and curvy. Guess what? It's also partly responsible for holding up the breasts.

In time, no matter how healthy your diet, of course, gravity will do its thing and your breasts will begin to sag—particularly if they are large and left to hang unsupported each day. Pregnancy and breastfeeding add to the problem when the breasts swell one or two cup sizes. Many women think that wearing a supportive bra during and after pregnancy will be enough to prevent sagging. Wearing a bra certainly helps, but as with everything else we've discussed, firm breasts have more to do with nutrition and muscular support.

Breast Anatomy

Breasts consist of fat, blood and lymph vessels, lobules, milk ducts (your mammary glands), lymph nodes, ligaments, and connective tissue. The size of your breasts is directly related to the amount of fat you store in your chest. What holds them up is the connective tissue, ligaments, and muscle—specifically the thick, fan-shaped pectoralis major muscle under the breasts.

During pregnancy, glucocorticoid hormones can cause the connective tissue around the breast to weaken. During lactation, the breast tissues are repeatedly stretched when the woman becomes engorged. After weaning, hormonal changes can cause the milk glands to atrophy somewhat. All of these factors may result in the appearance of looser skin. But much like your abdomen, the skin on your breasts requires time to firm up after the baby is born. Eating appropriately to maintain collagen and balanced hormones, and keeping the pectoral muscles strong are your best steps towards repairing, or even preventing, this problem.

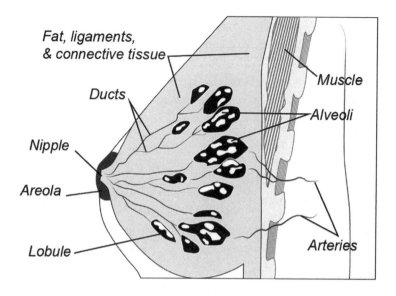

The Three Pillars of Breast Support

- Collagen building nutrients
- Muscular support
- Hormone balance

Improve Breast Firmness with Nutrition

To maintain and improve breast firmness, eat the nutrients necessary to build strong collagen. The dietary guidelines found in chapter 12 will strengthen the network of collagen and elastin fibers holding up the breasts. Additionally, it is equally important to eat a diet that encourages healthy hormone balance.

Improve Breast Firmness with Hormone Balance

As you will learn in Part III, hormone balance, just like nutritional deficiencies, affects the way we look on the outside. It is the key to maintaining collagen, storing fat in the breasts, and preventing glandular atrophy.

Remember that glucocorticoids inhibit healthy collagen production and that you can lower glucocorticoids by reducing stress and avoiding toxic and refined foods. Adequate progesterone levels also play a role in keeping corticosteroids under control.

Both estrogen and progesterone improve collagen production. In nursing and menopausal women, these hormones can be low. In some women androgens take their place. Progesterone also stimulates fat storage in the breast, whereas estrogen causes fat storage around the hips and thighs. Hence, balancing the ratio of progesterone and estrogen is important for maintaining and rebuilding breast firmness and size. Lowering estrogen by reducing exposure to chemicals and by balancing blood sugar levels will help to balance the hormones. You can help reduce estrogen dominance by applying a progesterone cream, but you should wait until after your pregnancy and breastfeeding have ended.

Improve Breast Appearance with Exercise

The breasts sit over the pectoralis major muscle but are not directly attached to it. This means that strengthening the muscle isn't going to lift up the breasts, but certain exercises—push-ups, modified push-ups (with knees on the ground), and chest presses—can add fullness and support and generally improve their appearance.

Vaginal Elasticity

The vagina is an elastic tract. It is designed to hold a penis, then stretch for a baby, then contract back to its previous size. The walls of the vagina are thick muscles composed of two layers: a weaker internal layer and a strong external layer. Covering these muscles is a sheath of connective tissue. Both strong muscle tone and collagen contribute to the tightness and elasticity of the vagina.

After childbirth the vagina will usually retract to its pre-pregnancy size, though it takes some time. There are a couple of factors that may hinder this process, however: vaginal dryness and weak pelvic floor muscles. These are common during and shortly after pregnancy.

Vaginal Dryness

Vaginal lubrication is important. For one thing, the wetness of the vagina is what makes it so elastic, allowing it to expand and retract more easily. This is because the collagen and elastin fibers are stronger when they are moist.

Vaginal dryness, on the other hand, not only hinders expansion and retraction, it can make sex uncomfortable and lead to vaginal and urinary tract infections.

Symptoms of vaginal dryness include:

- Burning during urination
- Pain during intercourse
- Light bleeding during intercourse
- Vaginal soreness
- Itching or burning sensations

Low estrogen—or estrogen disproportionately low in relation to progesterone—can cause vaginal dryness. Estrogen drops dramatically after delivery and stays low during lactation. It also drops dramatically as menopause approaches. Women with a low body fat ratio or who eat low fat diets can also have low estrogen. A woman in any of these situations can experience vaginal dryness.

Estrogen and progesterone exist in a delicate balance that can be easily maintained with a healthy diet and lifestyle. These two hormones are opposites and yet they complement each other; estrogen agitates and progesterone calms. When progesterone gets too low, estrogen can become dominant, and this results in a host of symptoms, including vaginal dryness. Additionally, progesterone is a precursor to estrogen, so if progesterone drops, estrogen can eventually drop too. At this point, a woman will miss the benefits of both hormones and the body will suffer in many ways. It is critical to maintain this balance to keep the vagina lubricated. Eating the diet outlined in this book will help, and, in the short term, there are a few options, including vaginal stimulation and the use of vaginal lubricants. According to Julia Schlam Edelmen, author of *Menopause Matters*, "Intercourse or masturbation twice a week maintains vaginal lubrication and vaginal health."

Ways to Increase Vaginal Lubrication

- Include fat and cholesterol in your diet (cholesterol is needed to produce estrogen)
- Bio-identical progesterone cream
- Stress management
- Reduced exposure to xenoestrogens
- Frequent sex or masturbation
- Natural water-based lubricants
- Avoid douching

Pelvic Floor Muscles

Strong pelvic floor muscles improve your sex life, help prevent incontinence, and support your other reproductive organs. There's muscle beneath the vagina's connective tissue layer, which needs to be toned, just like your abs. Pregnancy is often blamed for stretching out the pelvic floor muscles. While they do get weaker and looser, proper exercises after childbirth will firm them up. Many a pelvic prolapse (pelvic organs herniated through the vagina) could be avoided with strong pelvic muscles.

Kegel Exercises

Core exercises and everyday things like laughing, screaming, and singing keep your pelvic floor muscles toned, but for extra help you need Kegel exercises, which target those muscles specifically.

Women who work out and eat a diet high in collagen-building materials may never need to do these exercises. However, if you are lax in either of these areas, Kegels will strengthen the pelvic floor and prepare you for moving on to more rigorous core work.

How to do Kegel Exercises

1. **Locate the right muscles**—Kegel exercises are easy once you locate the correct muscles, which can take a little practice. The pelvic floor muscles are what you use to stop yourself from peeing. You can identify them by controlling your urine flow a couple of times.

2. **Practice**—Now that you've found the muscles, do the exercises with an empty bladder while sitting or lying down. If you feel the vagina and anus tighten and your buttocks and abdomen are relaxed, you're doing it correctly. In the beginning it may be difficult to hold the contraction for long. Start out by holding for 3-4 seconds, then relax for 3-4 seconds. Repeat 4 or 5 times.

3. **The routine**—Work up to keeping the muscles contracted for 10 seconds at a time, then relaxing for 10 seconds. Repeat 10 to 15 times per session and do 3 sessions per day. These exercises are inconspicuous and take only a few minutes; in other words, you can do them anywhere—at your desk, standing in line at the grocery store, or driving to work.

CHAPTER 12

Foods and Supplements to Support Connective Tissue

A traditional diet brings the hormones back into balance and reverses nutritional deficiencies—the two elements most responsible for preventing and repairing connective tissue damage. In order be successful at making these changes in our bodies, we must get serious about eating nutrient-dense foods and avoiding those lacking in nutrients—i.e., all of the refined and chemically altered products in abundance today. Junk food disrupts hormone balance; each time we substitute real food for fake food, we lose the opportunity to absorb and utilize supportive nutrients.

Many people think they can just eat whatever they want as long as they take daily supplements. And while it's true that very high quality supplements can help in restoring what our modern diets lack, they are not a magic bullet. Supplements fall short when digestion is impaired, for example, and when the supplements are synthetic or incomplete (you must choose them carefully). Whole foods offer the widest spectrum of nutrients, something that is not captured in a pill. Nevertheless, if local and clean sources of the foods are not available or if additional support is necessary, some of the following collagen-building nutrients may be taken in supplement form.

Keep in mind that connective tissue is regenerated slowly. Just as you wouldn't expect a broken bone to heal in a week or two, you shouldn't expect to quickly regenerate new collagen. Healing the body from within requires time and patience, but the rewards are profound and lasting.

Star Collagen Building Nutrients

The Building Blocks
Collagen is a protein that contains significant amounts of hydroxyproline and hydroxylysine. These amino acids are abundant in animal foods. While the body can manufacture these amino acids on its own, it is believed that

consumption of foods containing proline and lysine will contribute to collagen formation.

* **Proline and Lysine**—The class of extracellular macromolecules that make up our connective tissue are the proteins, such as collagen, which is found in abundance in the connective tissue. Collagen fibers are made up of the amino acids hydroxylysine and hydroxyproline.

From food	As a supplement
Proline and lysine are primarily found in animal protein. Catfish, chicken, and bone broth are good sources of lysine. Egg whites and gelatin-rich broths are particularly high in proline.	Probably the best supplement for proline and lysine is gelatin. When you don't have a pot of gelatin-rich broth ready, consider supplementing with gelatin. Great Lakes Gelatin is a trusted brand of both beef and porcine gelatin.

* **Glucosamine**—Much of the extracellular matrix is composed of substances that are converted from glucosamine. While the body does produce its own glucosamine, it may not be enough to repair extensive damage.

From food	As a supplement
Broth made from the bones of any animal or fish, or from egg and crustacean's shells, are high in a wide spectrum of glucosamine.	You may take glucosamine as a supplement at 1000 to 2000 mg/day, but it does not offer the full spectrum of tissue-repairing compounds found in broth.

Metabolism of Collagen Building Materials—So many women ask me why bone broth doesn't seem to be helping with their joint and skin problems. It may because they are not properly preparing the broth—I describe the proper method of broth preparation at the end of this chapter—but it also may be because they are missing the additional nutrients that help metabolize the building blocks of connective tissue; if they are missing, the bone broth and egg whites won't do you any good.

- **Vitamin A** regulates the production of the fibroblasts critical for synthesizing new collagen. Concentrate on getting your Vitamin A from animal sources; the synthesis from beta-carotene (plant sources) is unreliable at best.

From food	As a supplement
Liver, salmon, eggs, and butter are excellent sources of Vitamin A.	The Vitamin A found in high concentrations in cod liver oil is naturally occurring and considered safe.

- **Vitamin C** is necessary for protein synthesis, including the protein collagen. More Vitamin C is needed in high carbohydrate diets and during times of stress, so you should consider adding a supplement in addition to food.

From food	As a supplement
Citrus, peppers, and berries are a great source of Vitamin C, as is beef, broccoli, and chicken liver.	Supplemental Vitamin C is considered by most to be safe and effective. Take up to 2000 mg spaced throughout the day.

- **B Vitamins** aid in metabolizing glucosamine, amino acids, and EFAs into connective tissue.

From food	As a supplement
Fermented foods contain B Vitamins and a healthy gut produces them as well. They can also be found in milk, liver, nuts, leafy greens, and fruit.	Many of the B Vitamins sold are synthetic and come with side effects so a whole foods complex is best. Mega Food is one that uses folate instead of folic acid, the synthetic form of folate.

+ **Zinc** is necessary for cellular repair. It also helps boost the immune system and aids in wound healing. If you get sick often, or have skin problems, you are almost certainly deficient in zinc. Digestive problems can impair zinc absorption as can the phytates found in grains and legumes.

From food	As a supplement
The food with the highest concentration is oysters. Other healthy sources include chicken, nuts, crab, and red meat.	If oysters don't appeal to you or they are not available where you live, you can supplement with 15mg/day. Chelated zinc is often better absorbed than other varieties.

+ **Iron** plays a key role in metabolizing collagen. It also helps to carry oxygen to all of the cells in the body. Oxygen is most critical for the heart and other internal organs, so the body will always sacrifice the skin to maintain these vital organs. Menopausal women may have no need for iron supplementation, but women with heavy periods, pregnant women, women who have just given birth, or anyone with bleeding ulcers or impaired digestion might benefit from it. If you are not postmenopausal, make sure you get 18mg/day from food or otherwise. A pregnant woman's need for iron nearly doubles. The Recommended Dietary Allowance (RDA) for iron for pregnant women is 27 mg/day.

From food	As a supplement
The food with the highest concentration of iron is liver from chicken, then beef. Oysters, red meat, tuna, super dark chocolate, and spinach are also good sources.	Excessive iron can be very toxic and contribute to bacterial imbalance in the gut so take iron supplements as a last resort, when food sources aren't available.

Antioxidants For Preventing Oxidative Damage—Free radicals destroy everything in their path. Antioxidants neutralize these little hell raisers. There is evidence that in order for the body to work optimally in our toxic, stressful modern world, an antioxidant supplement should be a mainstay.

♦ **Antioxidant Cocktail**—Antioxidant rich foods should be eaten as vegetable and fruit salads throughout every day.

From food	As a supplement
Antioxidants are found in deeply pigmented foods such as berries, tea, dark chocolate, and oranges. They are easily destroyed, so eat them raw or barely cooked.	There are many options available on the market from super food powders to pills and tablets.

♦ **Bioflavonoids**—Vitamin C is a powerful antioxidant. But in order for the body to best utilize Vitamin C, it needs bioflavonoids.

From food	As a supplement
Vitamin C and bioflavonoids are found together in all citrus fruits, organ meats, and red peppers, among many other fruits and vegetables.	Rose hips and bioflavonoid combinations are sold in supplement form, but many Vitamin C supplements already contain them.

Anti-inflammatories—Inflammation causes disease, and the factors contributing to inflammation are everywhere you look: stress, excess body fat, processed foods, toxins, and even nutritional deficiencies. In order to calm the inflammation in our bodies and provide the best opportunity to heal, we must eat anti-inflammatory foods like fruits, vegetables, and seafood.

♦ **Anti-inflammatory cocktail**—Alpha lipoic acid (ALA), bromelain, ginger, resveratrol, turmeric, flaxseed oil, borage oil, evening primrose oil, fish oil, quercetin, and zinc are potent anti-inflammatories.

From food	As a supplement
ALA is found in broccoli and spinach; bromelain is found in pineapple; resveratrol is in the skin of red grapes and in red wine; quercetin is a bioflavonoid found in onions and apple peels.	All of these compounds are available as supplements.

- **Green Tea and Cherries**—Meet your new friends, *catechins* and *anthocyanidins*. Catechins help prevent the breakdown of collagen; anthocyanidins help the fibers link together. Green tea is high in catechins and deeply pigmented fruits like cherries and blueberries are high in anthocyanidins.

From food	As a supplement
For the most powerful nutritional punch, drink high quality whole leaf teas. Cherries and blueberries can be very high in pesticides so always go organic.	While it is probably unnecessary to take these as supplements if you are drinking tea and eating berries, they are available.

Other Important Nutrients

- **Lecithin**—When cell walls lack lecithin—the name for a group of fatty substances occurring in animal tissue—they can become damaged and weak. When cell walls are weak, they leak water. Dehydrated cells lead to damaged connective tissue.

From food	As a supplement
All of the lecithin you need for the day comes from a single egg yolk. If you don't eat eggs, you can also get lecithin from liver, fish eggs, and brains. What? You don't eat brains? That's okay. Your body makes lecithin itself. If your liver is healthy and you produce adequate bile, you probably manufacture all you need.	Lecithin is available as a supplement. One tablespoon provides enough lecithin for collagen-building.

- **Dietary Fat**—These fats not only play a huge role in the integrity of every cell, they carry the important skin nutrients Vitamins A, D, and E. Saturated fats provide the building blocks for hormones and are important for mineral absorption.

From food	As a supplement
Butter, beef, and coconut oil contain saturated fats. Monounsaturated fats are found in olives and macadamia nuts. Generally, you don't need to worry about obtaining polyunsaturated omega-6 oil; restricting them is more of a concern.	Saturated fat, so vilified in our culture, is the one thing not found in supplement form. But that's fine. The amount we need for healthy connective tissue far exceeds that which we could get in any pill anyway.

+ **Omega-3 fats**—The acids from these fats help build strong cell walls.

From food	As a supplement
All fatty fish are high in EFAs. Fish is very important during pregnancy and for overall health and should not be avoided. If you are concerned about mercury, choose smaller fish with shorter life spans. These include sardines, salmon, and mackerel.	If you are not eating fish two or three times per week, take 1000 to 2000 mg of cod liver oil per day.

+ **Magnesium**—Most Americans don't get enough of and it plays a critical role in cell function.

From food	As a supplement
Magnesium is abundant in fruits and vegetables, particularly oranges, spinach, almonds, and cocoa powder. Halibut is a good animal source of magnesium.	Magnesium citrate, the most common form of magnesium on the shelves, draws water into the bowels, so you may want to look for magnesium glycinate if you find that magnesium citrate disturbs your bowels.

How to Make Collagen Rich Bone Broth

Making bone broth is the easiest thing you can do in the kitchen. Just throw a few ingredients in a crock-pot, turn it on, and let it sit all day. The basic ingredients are clean water, chicken on the bone, some extra chicken parts like necks and backs or feet, a dash of vinegar, and salt. An acid, like vinegar, is essential for leeching out the minerals from the bones. If you don't like the smell or flavor of vinegar, you can try lemon juice. You will get a lot of value from the nutrients in the chicken's skin and the bones, but including the additional parts adds extra glucosamine and chondroitin. Both are great for connective tissue repair. I make chicken soup at least once a week in my slow cooker.

Simple Recipe for Chicken Bone Broth:

- 1 or 2 lbs. of free range chicken thighs
- 3 or 4 chicken feet
- A few chicken necks
- A handful of chicken livers
- Kelp powder or kombu for iodine
- 1 tbsp. sea salt
- 1 tbsp. vinegar (Important! The acid pulls the minerals from the bones)
- Herbs of your choice
- Water

Add collard greens, spinach, or chard for more minerals. In fact, throw in any other veggies you've got on hand. Put everything into a crock-pot, cover with water, and cook on low for the day.

A Quick Word About Water

Tap water contains everything from the neurotoxic fluoride to the traces of synthetic hormones, antibiotics, Rogaine, and anti-depressants people dump out in toilets. Tap water has been "purified"—i.e. it doesn't harbor bacteria, viruses, or dirt—but in most municipalities it is not free of harmful chemicals.

In ancient times (and in parts of the world today) water didn't have any contaminants from synthetic chemicals, but it did contain living organisms, dirt, and clay. Clean water is, of course, important for health. We definitely don't want to drink water contaminated with pathogenic bacteria. But because humans have always drunk water straight from the earth, purified water is not the most natural choice. For those of us who don't have a well in the backyard, we can add clays or mineral drops to bring some nutritional value back into the water.

Clays are both healing and mineral rich. Weston A. Price and others have noted that traditional peoples add small amounts of clay to their water for digestive health. A tablespoon of sodium bentonite or calcium bentonite clay, suitable for consumption, can be added to a glass of water. One glass on an empty stomach each day should be sufficient. Clays and mineral drops can be found in health food stores or online. One of the most popular edible varieties is green calcium bentonite clay, found in Death Valley, NV.

PART III

The Hormone Connection

Balanced hormones help to prevent and improve many of the ailments discussed in Part II by improving the fibroblast's ability to produce collagen. Hormones affect our moods, our growth, our creativity, our intelligence, and our fertility, for good and bad. When they are out of balance, any number of problems may result, from unwanted hair growth to fat deposits around the waist to the baby blues.

Eating responsibly is the best way to maintain our hormones' delicate balancing act, especially while pregnant. But some healthy food recommendations do more harm than good—like eating fruit. Fruit is healthier than cakes or ice cream, for sure, but eating too much of it can lead to unhealthy fluctuations in blood sugar. Pregnant women are advised to load up on veggies, but they can contain the harmful pesticides that contribute to hormonal imbalances. Pregnant women are instructed to consume more milk and cheese for strong bones, but the dairy they *choose might come from acidic, malnourished cows that are full of growth hormones and antibiotics. The meat of these animals also causes hormonal disruptions.*

In order to avoid many of the physical discomforts and unattractive symptoms associated with pregnancy, we must take care to ensure hormonal balance. I'm not going to lie to you: Balancing your hormones involves a radical change to your diet and lifestyle, and it won't be easy. But this is also where following the Primal path will yield the most deeply rewarding changes.

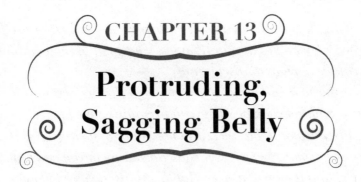

CHAPTER 13

Protruding, Sagging Belly

You just gave birth to a 7-plus pound baby, a huge pancake of tissue, and a deluge of fluids. That should just about flatten your stomach, right? So why is your pregnant-looking belly still hanging around weeks later?

Components of the Postpartum Belly

- Fat
- Water retention
- Slouched posture
- Enlarged uterus
- Weak abdominal muscles
- Stretched ligaments

Postpartum belly fat depends in part on how you ate while you were pregnant and in part on your hormones. Some of it can be blamed on weakened and stretched abdominal muscles. Some of it is water retention. (Immediate hormonal changes will prompt the body to start releasing those fluids in the form of urine, vaginal secretions, and sweat.) And some of it is the enlarged uterus and stretched-out ligaments. The good news: Most of the fat and bloating will be gone in about 6 weeks, if not sooner.

Many women are disappointed in the way they look after giving birth; they expect their belly to flatten out immediately. Other women are so busy with the new baby they don't even notice what they look like. The time spent nursing, napping, and figuring out your new life, might be enough to distract you, but once the little one starts sleeping through the night, you will probably start thinking a little more about how you look. By then you will have lost the excess water and will hopefully be exercising again. You may be impatient to get your old body back as soon as possible. There are a few things you can do to hasten the process.

Breastfeeding Shrinks the Uterus

After delivery, a mother begins to produce the hormone oxytocin, which is critical for developing the bond between mother and baby. This is the hormone that makes us so selfless even when we're sleep-deprived and physically and emotionally taxed. The constant presence of the baby triggers the brain to release oxytocin, but you can secrete even more if you breastfeed. There are great reasons to do that for the baby, and for you, too: Oxytocin is the hormone responsible for shrinking the uterus back to the size of a lemon.

As Kathleen Huggins, R.N., M.S., IBCLC, states in her book, *The Nursing Mother's Companion,* when a woman breastfeeds, the pituitary gland secretes oxytocin, which primarily acts on smooth muscle, contracting the sacs of milk in the breast. Contraction of the milk sacs causes milk to move to the front of the breast, making it available for baby. This is called the "letdown" reflex—an easily recognizable feeling. The uterus is also composed of smooth muscle tissue. With each feeding, oxytocin causes the smooth muscle in the uterus to contract as well, right back to its pre-pregnancy size. Even women who don't breastfeed secrete oxytocin; just having the baby causes its release. But breastfeeding motivates the pituitary to release a whole lot more. As soon as the baby starts to suckle, and every time thereafter for the next few weeks, the uterus shrinks a little more. By about week four, it should be back to its original size.

Belly Fat

How much weight you gain during pregnancy is based on a few things: your dietary and exercise choices, naturally, plus your stress levels. But your hormones are responsible for some of that weight, no matter what you do or don't do. And some of that fat gets deposited on the belly—possibly more than you saw before pregnancy.

Insulin levels are naturally elevated in a pregnant woman; that's how glucose is passed to the baby. But insulin increases the hormone androgen, which causes fat to be deposited in the midsection. In late pregnancy, extra cortisol is released to help prepare for labor. Cortisol, a stress hormone, also has a reputation for adding inches to the middle. After delivery, your hormones should return to normal and fat storage will decline and redistribute. But then comes breastfeeding; progesterone is naturally lower in the body during lactation, and estrogen and testosterone can easily become dominant. Because of this, breastfeeding mothers can find it nearly impossible to shed a single pound.

Saggy Belly Skin

Sagging skin on the abdomen can be related to the hormonal imbalances that weaken connective tissue and abdominal muscles. Additionally, if there is a lot of fat on the belly and the abdominal muscles are stretched thin, the skin has a big job to do holding it taut. This is when your belly needs a little TLC; the body's connective tissue must be strengthened and the fat burned.

Weak Abdominal Muscles

Our hormones are smart: They don't do more work than they have to. There are no hormones, for example, that *cause* the abdominal muscles to shrink back to their normal size and density. Now, smooth muscle is acted upon via hormones but skeletal muscle changes shape only through conscious contraction—in other words, we have to work at it. The good news is that, by nature, human beings are not sedentary. The bad news is that many human beings have become quite sedentary in modern times. If you've spent the last nine months barely lifting a finger (going against nature, in other words) your abdominal muscles have probably turned into pudding.

Weak abdominal muscles will create the illusion of a bigger belly. Any belly that has been stretched to full term is going to be weaker than usual. Of course, just how weak the muscles get depends on your level of activity during pregnancy. Maintaining an active lifestyle will help the abs stay strong, even without targeted exercises. But a few specific abdominal exercises during pregnancy can't hurt, and they will certainly make postpartum recovery easier.

Proper Alignment

Slouched posture makes your belly look bigger. In fact, much of the pooch you see in postpartum women (and in women in general) is a result of bad posture. I already went over alignment in chapter 10. Here I will explain something you probably think you know how to do already: stand up straight.

The typical postpartum posture is misaligned due to your growing belly, which shifts your body's center of gravity. During the latter half of pregnancy, the pelvis tilts forward and the pubic bone tips backward. This increases the curve of the lower spine. You may have noticed this is how fashion models stand when they want to look "sexy." The sexiness is debatable but it's definitely not healthy. The eventual response to this posture is a forward curve of the upper back and tipping of the neck; in addition, the belly pushes out and the chest caves in. After delivery, women must take extra care to realign the pelvis, neck, and upper back.

Proper alignment of the spine is the first step in conditioning the abdominals and making them look smaller. In fact, by simply standing up straight, you can eliminate half of your belly. But there are myriad benefits beyond that. By maintaining proper alignment you can:

- Avoid injuries
- Get the most out of each targeted abdominal exercise
- Reduce or eliminate back pain
- Improve digestion
- Increase blood flow
- Improve balance
- Ease emotional issues
- Increase flexibility

After the delivery of Evelyn, I began to work on alignment and posture for the first time in my life. It had remarkable effects on my body image, my mental health, digestive health, and physical comfort. In fact, it helped in the conditioning of all of my muscle groups.

The Jaw

Because I am a singer, I started with the alignment of my jaw. This is neglected in exercise books, and yet most people raised on nutrient-deficient diets need the help. Mineral deficiencies cause a change in the skeleton, starting with the face. The narrowing of the skeleton can cause misalignment of the spine, put pressure on the skull, and affect your moods. The pressure on the skull can be somewhat alleviated by relaxing the jaw and allowing it to hang freely, rather than tucking it back into the neck. This simple change can improve breathing through the nose and offer the face the appearance of a larger jaw. Since I sing, relaxing the jaw is essential for proper technique, but it is beneficial for everyone.

Discover Good Posture on the Floor

- **The Spine:** To find a neutral spine, lie on your back with knees bent and feet flat on the floor, arms by your side, palms flat on the floor. Place your feet a foot-and-a-half from your buttocks, and leave about four inches between your knees.

- **The Pelvis:** There are a couple of common mistakes we make when we lie on our backs. Either we hyperextend the spine or we push it all the way to the floor. Our aim here is a neutral spine. To find that relaxed position, rock your pelvis a few times to release any tension.

- **The Shoulders:** Between stress and the time we spend sitting in front of computer screens, most of our shoulders are tense even when we think they're relaxed. Check your shoulders for tension by rolling one shoulder up off the floor, taking care to leave the ribs and pelvis still. Now slide the shoulder blades down the back, moving the shoulders away from the ears. Repeat on the other side.

- **The Head:** Again, we're looking for neutral rotation. You don't want your chin tucked into your neck, nor do you want your chin pointing up towards the ceiling.

Bring Your New Posture to a Standing Position

Stand in front of a wall or mirror. Place the heels of your hands on the bony points of your hips and reach your index fingers diagonally toward your groin. Keep this area vertical to the wall. To find this ideal position, rotate your hips forward and back. Don't worry so much about how much curve is in the small of your back. Everyone has varying degrees of curvature; this is natural. Now, lengthen the spine upward, drop the shoulders down your back, and lift and drop the head so that your ears are directly above your shoulders. If you are doing this in front of a mirror, you should notice that you look longer and leaner already!

Gentle Exercises for Rebuilding the Core

How much will you need to do to strengthen your abdominals after the baby is born? That depends on how much or how little you did before and during your pregnancy.

A good way to tell if it's safe to resume your regular abdominal exercises is by checking the distance between your abdominis rectus muscles. To determine this, lie on your back, lift the head slightly, and place two fingers about an inch above the navel. If two fingers or less fit in the gap between the two muscles, then your connective tissue is in good shape and crunches probably won't harm you. If it is wider than two fingers, begin with the abdominal-splinting exercises we went over in chapter 10.

Transverse Abdominal Compressions

The transverse abdominal (TVA) muscles are essential for flattening the abs and strengthening the pelvic floor. Think of the TVAs as the deepest of the core muscles. You use the transverse abdominal muscles when you suck in your gut. Since the pelvic floor muscles engage simultaneously when the TVAs are used, working these muscles will also help strengthen the pelvic floor.

Most people favor other abdominal muscles, but the TVAs are easy to train. Best of all, these exercises can (and should) be done safely throughout and after pregnancy. They put no pressure on the rectus abdominis and are fine for women with diastasis recti.

Sit cross-legged on the floor, back straight. It helps to close your eyes and really concentrate on what you're doing. Now suck your navel towards your spine—not your ribs or your "six pack" (rectus abdominals), just your navel. If you place your hands on either side of your belly button, you should see your fingers move towards the heels of your feet. Hold this for 20 seconds. If your TVAs are strong, you should be able to hold this pose indefinitely. You can use this technique any time you want to make your belly appear slimmer. While doing this exercise, you should also feel your pelvic floor tightening slightly—not as much as when you are doing Kegels, but they are strengthening nevertheless.

Yoga for Rebuilding the Core

There are myriad abdominal exercises you can do but I prefer the gentle, effective, and safe poses of yoga for the early postpartum woman. In general, yoga is great for core strength but it also focuses on alignment. Doing yoga regularly and focusing on good form will undoubtedly firm your belly. Here are two of the easiest poses to do at home; both eliminate the need for regular crunches.

Begin these exercises as soon as any stiches have been removed and after incisions or tears begin to heal. Women who have kept up with abdominal conditioning should be able to hold these exercises longer than those who have not.

Plank Position

Get down on all fours, placing the palms of your hands and your knees on the floor. Your hands should be directly under the shoulders and your knees directly under the hips. Keep your back as flat as a tabletop with your elbows facing the back of the room. Remove the tension from your shoulders by sliding them down your back. Tuck your toes under and lift your knees up off of the floor. You should be holding up your weight with just your hands and toes. Imagine your body is as straight as a wood plank (thus the name of the pose); don't let your hips rise up. Hold this pose for 30 seconds or longer, inhaling and exhaling calmly. People with very strong abs can do this for two or three minutes, but it isn't easy.

Boat Pose

Begin by sitting up straight on the floor with your legs pressed together in front of you. If your abdominals are still very weak, start with the half boat pose: Bend your knees and place your hands on the backs of your thighs. Simultaneously lean back and lift your legs off the floor so that your shins are parallel with the floor.

If this is easy, go for full boat pose. Instead of bending your knees, stretch your legs out. Place your hands behind the head or, for a greater challenge, extend them directly in front of you. Simultaneously lift your straight legs and lean back, assuming a V position. Hold this pose for as long as you can, counting the seconds. Your goal should be 1 minute. Don't forget to breathe!

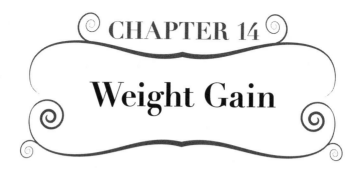

CHAPTER 14

Weight Gain

Pregnant women gain weight. It's normal and true for everyone no matter what part of the world they live in. But American women seem to gain more than women of other cultures. Why is that? For starters, their food options differ. The notion of what is healthy is also different. Furthermore, American women are generally advised to gain more weight than is necessary during pregnancy. That translates for a lot of us into eating (overeating in too many cases) unhealthy, weight-promoting foods.

Female Fat Storage

Females have a higher percentage of body fat than men. Sorry, that's just the way it is. This gender difference begins around age eight and revs up at adolescence, when the fat cells of girls begin increasing in size. By adolescence, those cells are increasing in number, too.

This extra fat, governed by hormones, is found mostly in the buttocks and thighs, which is difficult to shed. Unfair, perhaps, but it's for a good reason. We would be seriously compromising our femininity if we ditched this sex-specific fat. More importantly, the fat serves a reproductive purpose, acting as a reserve for the energy demands of lactation.

The female body is equipped to gear up for periods of scarcity by storing extra fat on the hips and thighs. This fat storage is great for the survival of the species, but some American doctors are taking the recommendation for pregnancy weight gain a little too far.

Pregnancy Weight Gain Recommendations in the 20th Century

In the 1930s, doctors told pregnant women to gain roughly 15 pounds during pregnancy. In the 1940s and 1950s, obstetricians bumped up the pounds to 20. Today, we are told to gain between 25 and 35 pounds, regardless of our build or weight before pregnancy (obese mothers are the exception).

Go ahead and Google it! A whole community of health writers has followed the herd. The most recent tables breaking down the distribution of weight gain report bigger numbers, too.

This is a little odd isn't it? Women haven't changed that much, and neither has the weight of carrying a baby.

The Actual Weight of Carrying a Baby

* Baby—8 lbs.
* Placenta – 1 ½lbs.
* Amniotic fluid – 2lbs.
* Increased size and weight of the uterus – 2 ½lbs.
* Larger breasts – 1lb.
* Blood volume – 3 ½lbs.

Total: 18 ½ lbs.

Add in some extra fat to carry the baby to term (unless the woman already has extra fat to begin with), which could equal several more pounds. A normal pregnancy, therefore, shouldn't require a weight gain of more than 19-23 pounds. So why are doctors now recommending a gain of up to 35 pounds? Let me count the ways:

* Many pregnant women think they're eating for two, which isn't the case at all. They're actually eating for 1 and about 1/10.
* Junk food is ubiquitous and addictive, especially when pregnant women are told to eat, eat, eat!
* Somewhere along the line exercise for pregnant women became taboo, which instigates the hormonal imbalances that encourage increased fat storage.

- The advice of doctors is to eat plenty of grains, fruits, dairy, and legumes, all while lowering fat—which is funny since all of those foods cause blood sugar to spike, and that leads to fat storage and cravings for more high-carb foods.

So what do you get, given all of the above? Scales adjusted for our fatter population. Add to that the fact that, when devising the new weight gain breakdown, the authors no long included half pounds; they rounded up to yield higher totals.

- Baby – 8 lbs.
- Placenta – 2-3lbs.
- Amniotic Fluid – 2-3lbs.
- Increased size and weight of the uterus – 2-5 lbs.
- Larger Breasts – 2-3 lbs.
- Blood volume – 4 lbs.

Our revised 21st century table adds up to 20-26 pounds. Plus, doctors now routinely recommend that pregnant women gain an additional 5-9 pounds in order to carry the baby to term and to ensure breastfeeding. That adds up to a total of 25-35 pounds for "healthy" pregnant women in the US.

This is odd because the weight of amniotic fluid hasn't changed, pregnant women's breasts aren't getting bigger, blood volume is the same, and a placenta is a placenta. So why the sudden difference in numbers? Well, either there is adipose tissue weighing down the placenta, greater blood volume for a greater-sized woman, and water retention in the breasts and amniotic fluid, or they're lying to us and nothing has changed but our acceptance of being fat.

I carried my first baby to term—41 weeks to be exact—and I produced enough breast milk to feed a whole nursery! I breastfed for 18 months. In total, I gained a little less than 18 pounds. So, let's see: How much weight do we really *need* to gain to have a healthy pregnancy, baby, and milk production? Not as much as they say we do.

Too Much Weight Gain Is Not Good

Gaining a little more fat than I did certainly isn't going to do any harm to mother or baby—I was very active while I was pregnant and quite strict about avoiding non-Paleo foods—but there is a limit if you want to keep both mother and baby in good health. Significant and rapid weight gain causes a disruption of hormones and acts as a storage place for toxins. Being heavy causes undue stress on the joints and puts pressure on the abdomen, contributing to diastasis recti. Excess fat feeds inflammation on a cellular level and contributes to fatigue and lack of coordination. Researchers in Finland found that women who gain excess weight during pregnancy are at a higher risk of developing breast cancer. Clearly, excess fat on our bodies is harmful to us, and as it turns out it's also harmful to the baby.

The Risks for Heavier Babies

A 2010 study of 513,501 mothers and 1,164,750 of their children born across a 15-year span assessed maternal and infant weight for women with more than one child. Researchers, led by David Ludwig, director of the obesity program at Children's Hospital Boston, looked at the differences and similarities in birth weight based on maternal weight rather than genetics. They found that heavier women do indeed have heavier babies and that this outcome is independent of genetics. For every kilogram gained during pregnancy, the baby's weight increased by about 9.5 grams, according to the analysis published in *The Lancet*.

Heavier babies are notoriously more difficult to birth. The excess fat puts pressure on the baby's joints and may lead to joint problems later in life.

Passing On Obesity, Cancer, and Asthma

By eating too much during pregnancy you may saddle your child with problems beyond weight. As Dr. Ludwig reported in the study above, "Since high birth weight…increases risk for obesity and diseases such as cancer and asthma later in life, these findings have important implications for general public health."

Hormonal Imprinting

As you know by now, weight gain causes a disruption in your hormone balance. And since you are sharing your body with your baby, he or she will inherit those imbalances and suffer the consequences well into adolescence and adulthood.

Hormonal imprinting, as it is called, affects how a child responds to hormones for the rest of its life. Lack of iodine in the mother's diet, for example, impacts the thyroid of a developing fetus. A mother who contributes to her own estrogen imbalance by gaining too much weight or eating too much sugar will also adversely affect her child. For this reason, it's important to eat consciously before and during your pregnancy. Think of it not as eating for two, but *living* for two.

Causes of Weight Gain

It's pretty clear that overeating leads to weight gain. But the types of foods we overeat matter as well. Processed foods cause hormonal disruptions, nutrient deficiencies, inflammation, changes in our brain chemistry, and altered gut ecology. When this happens losing weight can become difficult or almost impossible.

Hormones

When hormones are out of balance, our bodies respond in all sorts of unpleasant ways. One is by going into fat storage mode. Many women (and men) excuse weight gain by blaming it on their hormones, Yes, hormones out of balance can cause weight gain, only guess who is primarily responsible for those imbalances? You are the one with the power to cause damage, but you also are the one with the power to repair it.

Some of the hormones that can contribute to excess weight gain during pregnancy include:

+ **Cortisol**—This plays many roles in the body but is best known as the hormone behind fight-or-flight syndrome. In times of danger or extreme stress cortisol is secreted to help us get to safety. It does this by triggering the release of sugar, which is very helpful when we're actually in trouble. When that happens, the extra energy is used up in flight so there's no weight gain. But modern stress comes in less obviously life threatening forms: while we're sitting in our cars getting angry about traffic, or in our office chairs worrying about deadlines. In these cases, the extra energy is not being used up, so it gets stored as fat. The long-term problem with this is that chronically elevated cortisol leads to chronically elevated blood sugar, and that's because cortisol's other function is to suppress insulin.

+ **Ghrelin**—Since insulin is needed by cells to metabolize sugar, elevated blood sugar combined with suppressed insulin starves the cells of the necessary glucose. This causes the body to release excess ghrelin—the hormone that makes us feel hungry. If you've ever wondered why you are still fiercely craving food when you are clearly full, you probably have excess ghrelin.

✦ **Leptin**—This is the hormone responsible for making us feel full. When we are healthy, leptin works to suppress appetite and speed up the metabolism after a meal, or when the body recognizes it has had too much nutrition. Leptin helps us to effortlessly regulate our weight. When we gain a few pounds, it comes to the rescue, suppressing our appetite so that we can easily lose the extra pounds. When leptin receptors are unresponsive (a condition called leptin resistance), our desire for food remains active. Leptin resistance is caused both by what we eat and what we don't. In order to regain sensitivity to leptin, we need to reduce inflammation.

Inflammation

Inflammation is at the root of many diseases, including arthritis, asthma, allergies, and colitis. It is now recognized as the root of many cases of obesity as well. Factors such as a poor diet, environmental toxins, stress, and lack of exercise all trigger an inflammatory response.

Inflammation contributes to fat storage by making the body resistant to leptin, cortisol, and insulin, making it very difficult to lose weight. According to Dr. Leo Galland, author of *The Fat Resistance Diet*, inflammation triggers leptin resistance because of the body's natural response to inflammation.

How Inflammation Works

When we injure ourselves—break an arm, get a cut or infection—our immune systems come to the rescue with white blood cells. The site gets swollen, red, and hot due to the extra white cells and increase in blood flow. While inflammation can be uncomfortable, it helps to heal the infection or injury.

I have described acute inflammation—localized inflammation obvious to the eye. But it clearly has a counterbalance or you'd have evidence of every cut and scrape from childhood. The counterbalance is anti-inflammatory chemicals, which the body sends out to call off the rescue mission. In a world where injury and infection are not the norm, this process is functional, but in a world such as ours, where inflammatory assaults are as common as wind blowing through the trees, it's not so good.

Lack of exercise, poor diet, toxins, stress, and obesity cause what has come to be known as chronic inflammation, or inflammation which is always turned on. In a simpler, healthier world, inflammation was occasional; now it is constant and systemic.

Inflammation Causes Leptin Resistance

The consequence of this new environment goes beyond just the side effects of the inflammation itself. Our bodies must also deal with the regular onslaught of anti-inflammatory chemicals, which, according to Dr. Galland, disrupt the body's response to leptin. Chronic inflammation leads to leptin resistance.

Taking care to reduce the inflammation caused by our environment will help regulate weight. Eating anti-inflammatory foods will aid in calming the inflammation already present in the system, in addition to protecting the body from further inflammation. Avoiding certain inherently inflammatory foods—e.g, wheat, sugar, processed vegetable oils, an excess of omega 6 oils like corn, sunflower, and soybean—will also help to prevent and heal chronic inflammation.

Reducing inflammation isn't just good for your weight. In general, following these principles will not only improve your ability (and your child's ability) to fight infections, it will take you a long way towards beauty, longevity, and happiness.

Obesity's Role in Inflammation

Adipose tissue itself causes inflammation. Fat cells actually produce their own hormones. The bigger these fat cells get (i.e., the fatter a person becomes) the more inflammatory hormones—called adipokines—the fat cells will produce.

The two specific adipokines produced by fat cells are TNF-alpha and IL-6. TNF-alpha is known for causing the tissue damage and pain that accompanies rheumatoid arthritis, as well as other autoimmune disorders. TNF is also a major contributor to insulin resistance. Not only do fat cells produce these hormones, our immune systems do too. You don't *have* to be obese or overweight to suffer from these conditions, but obesity certainly contributes to and exacerbates the problem.

Producing excess adipokines isn't the only harm our enlarged fat cells are doing. The fat cells of an obese person are kind of like an overblown balloon. When a balloon gets overfilled, the latex tears. This is the same for fat cells. The membrane of a fat cell can only expand so much before its integrity is compromised. In the body, these tears are injuries and so the immune system is called in for repair. When fat cells break, white blood cells called macrophages—the garbage collectors of the immune system—are sent in for cleanup duty. While the macrophages are busy, they are also dropping off inflammatory chemicals. The presence of these chemicals tells the cells to release anti-inflammatory chemicals in response. These are the chemicals—called SOCS (suppressors of cytokine signaling)—that interfere with leptin sensitivity.

If you find yourself overeating for a period or eating a highly inflammatory diet, inflammation and weight gain can ensue. And, unfortunately, both of those, even if temporary, cause even more inflammation and weight gain. Eventually this gets out of control as leptin resistance produces a vicious cycle of fat storage and inflammation. At this point a person may find that no diet or amount of exercising or calorie-counting helps to drop the weight. The only feasible route will be to restore leptin sensitivity through an anti-inflammatory diet and healthy lifestyle choices.

Anti-inflammatory Foods

* Vegetables, especially onions, garlic, and dark leafy greens.

* Spices such as cayenne and turmeric

* Black and green teas

* Fruits, especially deeply pigmented fruits like cherries and berries

* Fish and cod liver oil

Nutritional Deficiencies and Weight Gain

Deficiency in any of the following nutrients can also explain weight gain:

* **Vitamin D** deficiency is extremely common in the US, thanks in part to the use of sunscreen. Despite the recommendations to cover up any time you go outside, you should expose a large part of your body to UVB rays for 30 minutes a couple of times a week. After that, you are welcome to put the sunscreen on to avoid too much exposure. (For more on this, go to chapter 17.)

* **Iodine** deficiency can contribute to hypothyroidism, which is sometimes responsible for weight gain.

* **B Vitamins** boost metabolism, so when they are lacking, our metabolism slows down, leading to weight gain.

* **Vitamin C** helps convert glucose to energy, which prevents the glucose from getting stored as fat. Without enough Vitamin C, the starches and sugars we eat go right to our fat cells.

* **Chromium** deficiency is rare, but adding it to the diet can help balance blood sugar, reduce cravings, and maintain better insulin control.

+ **Magnesium** deficiency is very common and plays a big role in metabolizing carbs.

Damaged Gut

Our stomach and intestines contain trillions (yes, trillions!) of microbes, including bacteria and yeasts. Researchers are beginning to understand that the human being has a symbiotic relationship with these creatures and that without them we are more susceptible to a multitude of modern diseases. Unfortunately, our gut microbes have been decreasing in the last few decades, and that's having a devastating effect on our health.

Jeffery Gordon, Director of Washington University's Center for Genome Sciences, and his team have shown that people of normal weight favor a family of bacteria called *bacteroidetes*, while obese people have more *firmicutes*. His team was able to prove that gut microbes actually contribute to obesity. He found that "transplanting the gut microbiota from normal mice into germ-free recipients increases their body fat without any increase in food consumption."

What this means is that bacteria might actually be responsible for the amount of calories we absorb, with the bad bacteria somehow causing us to retain more. If this is true, two people could eat the same number of calories but absorb a different number. According to Paleo nutrition advocate Chris Kresser, a doctor in San Francisco, "Different species of bacteria seem to have different effects on appetite and metabolism." Studies suggest that certain strains of bacteria are actually responsible for the systemic inflammation that leads to obesity.

The microbial landscape of our gut can be altered and improved by eliminating edible toxins like antibiotics and packaged foods and by adding fermented and raw foods to the diet.

Cravings and Neurotransmitters

Imbalanced brain chemicals can lead to weight gain just like imbalanced hormones and an unhealthy gut can. A lack of certain neurotransmitters, for example, can cause us to crave certain foods to compensate for that lack. For example, an urge for hard candy, bread, or fruit on its own (not combined with protein or fat) signifies a need for serotonin. Serotonin is released in response to the tryptophan surge after consuming carbohydrates alone.

Anxious women often go for fatty sweet foods—a piece of coconut cream pie or a chewy chocolate chip cookie—because it triggers the release of dopamine. It is the food's texture, taste, and aroma—its "pleasurability"—that triggers the release, so everyone has their own favorite fix. These neurotransmitters are more potent during pregnancy, which explains the midnight hankering for a bowl of ice cream.

Since our body is a well-designed machine that, when left alone, would only do what's best for itself, there is a mechanism for craving the nutrients we *truly* need. That explains why a healthy woman is more likely to go for a clean diet; she can trust the language of her desires better than the woman who subsists on junk food. If you are pregnant and have indulged in an unhealthy diet, don't give in to cravings. Instead, reprogram your body by eating the foods you truly need.

Weight Loss Strategies

In a nutshell, no matter what you do, you'll lose weight or avoid gaining it when you trade processed foods for fresh and unprocessed foods. Ideally, you will make the switch before you get pregnant, and, if you're overweight, lose the excess pounds before you conceive. There are women who don't see the point in losing weight if they trying to conceive anyway, but this is a mistake. If you don't improve your health before you get pregnant, you risk passing on your own toxicity and inflammation to your child.

The Dangers of Detoxing While Pregnant and Breastfeeding
No matter what stage you're in—thinking about getting pregnant, pregnant, postpartum—there is an appropriate weight strategy for you. If you're not pregnant yet, get to work achieving your optimum weight, establish a healthy gut and hormone balance, and work on nutrient reserves. If you're pregnant or breastfeeding, however, significant weight loss should not be your goal—a side effect of your improved diet perhaps, but not a goal.

Rapid weight loss usually results from some kind of dietary restriction, either from lowering carbohydrates or fat. A healthy eating and exercise strategy will inevitably induce some amount of weight loss, but postpone any further restrictions until breastfeeding has ceased. This is because weight loss induces detoxification and you don't want to deliberately mobilize toxins while still feeding your baby. As long as those toxins sit tight in your fat cells, you can rest assured the baby won't be harmed by them.

A Note on Dieting While Pregnant
If you are already plump, you probably don't need to gain more than the minimum of 18 ½ pounds—maybe even less. You don't need to focus on gaining

any extra weight for healthy hormonal balance. If you are obese to begin with, you might not want to gain any weight at all. Researchers are in the process of evaluating the effects of zero weight gain while pregnant. Obviously, this translates to an overall fat loss. Over nine months, the mother is going to lose 18 pounds. She should not do this deliberately through calorie restriction; she should do it by maintaining a nutrient-dense diet. The boost in nutrition will help to balance her hormones and reduce inflammation, both of which will result in effortless weight loss. The most important thing is to be sure that both mother and baby are constantly supplied with sufficient nutrients.

Ketones and Carbohydrate Restriction

Ketones are the compounds produced when fat is burned for energy, whether the fat comes from the diet or from the body itself. Some people are concerned that they are harmful to a fetus. A handful of researchers surmise that ketones cause a lowered IQ, but these findings are controversial because the conclusions were drawn from research from an unrelated study on diabetic pregnant women. There is absolutely no way to know if the ketones were actually responsible for their findings.

Looking at it from an evolutionary perspective, it would seem that the ketones themselves are probably not to blame. The conditions necessary to produce ketones—e.g., occasional skipped meals, extended length between meals, and lower carbohydrate intake—would have been common throughout human history. It is likely that there were other factors that caused the cognitive difficulties, such as diabetes, possibly obesity, or any number of other unobserved factors.

Nevertheless, there has been little to no research on pregnant women eating low carb diets. Whether they are suitable or harmful to adults and their babies remains to be seen.

Get Nutrients and Absorb Them

Certain nutrients can contribute to weight loss while the lack of them can contribute to weight gain. Depending on your own gut health, however, adding these nutrients may not do you much good. You can eat a nutrient-dense diet for years, but if you don't absorb the nutrients that you eat you lose any benefit. Avoiding all of the foods which you are sensitive to or which otherwise impair your digestion will dramatically improve health and weight loss.

Establish a Healthy Gut Ecology

Rebuilding gut flora is essential for human health but it isn't always easy in the modern world; a lot of those necessary microbes are being driven to extinction by our sterile and toxic diets and lifestyles. By reducing toxic exposure, eliminating sterile packaged foods, by getting our hands dirty in nature, and never using anti-bacterial soap, we can start to rebuild what we have lost, lose weight, and get healthy again. Begin with these steps:

Ways to Improve Gut Health

- Stop using birth control and NSAIDs
- Stop using antibiotics
- Treat pathogens such as parasites with herbs (postpone if pregnant)
- Take a probiotic and eat fermented foods
- Eliminate sugar
- Eat more fermentable, soluble fibers
- Avoid dietary toxins and industrial seed oils
- Reduce stress

Reduce Inflammation

Here are some steps to reduce inflammation:

- **Exercise**—Engage in some form of physical activity every day.
- **Oils**—Use anti-inflammatory oils like olive, flax, coconut, fish, and CLA (conjugated linoleic acid) from grass fed beef.
- **Phytonutrients**—Include foods rich in phytonutrients (fruits, vegetables, nuts, and teas).
- **Eliminate inflammatory foods**—Wheat, processed oils, and sugar should be removed.

De-stress

In addition to a leaky gut, stress causes the release of hormones like cortisol, which leads to fat storage.

Stress Relief Techniques:

- Talking with a therapist
- Meditation
- Yoga
- Deep breathing
- Guided imagery
- Exercise

- Massage
- Sleep; a 2004 study at the University of Wisconsin-Madison revealed that subjects who slept less had lower levels of leptin and higher levels of ghrelin.

Move Your Body

Without exercise, gut health suffers, hormone balance suffers, sleep patterns suffer, the elimination of toxins is stalled, and you cannot achieve optimal health. Despite what some believe, you will not lose weight with exercise alone, but it is an essential part of any weight loss strategy.

Combined Efforts Work Best

It takes time to repair the damage we have done to ourselves. Adding supplements or special foods to a healthy diet and trying to maintain a low stress lifestyle will help speed up the process. Just taking supplements, however, or simply getting a walk in every day won't be enough. Losing weight and improving health and the quality of your life is a multi-tiered process. But here's the payoff: You will be a mom that looks good naked!

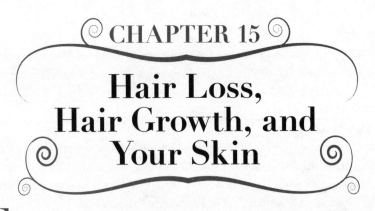

CHAPTER 15

Hair Loss, Hair Growth, and Your Skin

The color, texture, and thickness of our hair is determined by genetics, the food we eat, and our hormones. Genetics is the biggest influence when it comes to our hair. No matter how healthy I am and no matter how many hair growth vitamins I take, I will never have thick, abundant, curly hair. That's just not in my genes. Conversely, many women who do have gorgeous hair do not eat the foods necessary to maintain it. Their strong genes have them covered in the hair department.

But even if we weren't well-endowed from childhood, each of us can make the most of our genetic potential and have the best version of the hair we were programmed to have. We can eat a Primal diet, or keep our hormones balanced. Or we can get pregnant. Turns out pregnancy can have a profoundly positive effect on hair.

The Luscious Locks of the Pregnant Woman

Thanks to the elevated hormones, hair can change for the better during pregnancy. For some women, the hair gets a little darker thanks to melanocyte-stimulating hormones (MSH), which promote the melanin-producing cells that give hair its color. Other women enjoy thicker hair thanks to estradiol, the hormone that prolongs the growth phase and prevents the normal process of shedding.

How Hair Growth Works

About 89 percent of our hair is actively growing. This is called the anagen phase, which usually lasts about six years. Another 1 percent of our hair is in the atrophy phase, meaning the hair stops growing but is not shed. That's because it's waiting for the telogen, or resting, phase, which is when the remaining 9 percent of hair is shed and replaced. Within a few months, the hairs in the telogen phase will fall out and fresh ones will take their place.

A normal head loses 100-300 hairs per day. That may seem like a lot, but it's actually not: We have a whopping 5 million hair follicles to play with. In fact, losing those few pieces each day is exactly what our hair needs to stay fresh and healthy looking.

How Hair Growth Changes During Pregnancy...

When a woman is pregnant, her resting phase slows dramatically. This begins just a few months into pregnancy. Since we're not losing as much hair, it will start to look fuller. Here's a conservative estimate of the number of extra hairs we hold onto each day over the course of four months: 120,000. For me at least, that looks like a decent chunk and, indeed, while pregnant my hair was fuller and longer than ever!

...And Then It All Falls Out

A fuller head of hair is attractive without a doubt, which should serve to make us feel pretty while we're pregnant. Unfortunately, once our bodies are back to normal, we lose the benefit.

When estrogen levels decline, the length of the resting phase returns to normal. For a time, you might wonder if there's something wrong with you, but this hair loss is normal and makes sense: there are now more hairs that will be entering the resting phase than there were before you got pregnant. Within a few months, all those extras will fall out. Remember that only 15 percent of hair is in the resting phase at any given time. Since 100 percent of your hair is now a bigger number than it used to be, 15 percent of your hair is also a bigger number than it used to be. Hence you've got more hair falling out. It can take six months for this process to complete, so in the meantime get yourself a drain cover and vacuum regularly.

Hormonal Hairs

Pregnant women can also develop more hair where they *don't* want it: the chin, breasts, navel, and upper lip.

While some of this is normal—pregnant means you're pumped up with more hormones than you will experience during the rest of your life—excess hair can also be a sign of a slight or major hormonal imbalance, depending on the degree of growth and if it is in combination with other symptoms.

Dark Hairs

Some of the elevated hormones during pregnancy have the effect of boosting sebum, or skin oil. They can also darken hair in unwanted places. A few such hairs are fine and can be easily tweezed. When they become excessive, however, they can signify excessive levels of androgens, the so-called male hormones. (It's normal for a woman's body to produce and circulate small amounts of androgens.)

Excess androgen production afflicts pregnant women and women with hormonal disorders. In fact, it is the women who have had this problem before conceiving who will see it magnified during pregnancy. (But not always! If you resolve the hormonal imbalances before pregnancy, they will not magically reappear during pregnancy. I resolved my androgen imbalances years ago and none of it resurfaced while I was pregnant.)

Dark hormonal hairs are caused when the skin reacts to testosterone on the skin. Excess testosterone production is something that women with Polycystic Ovary Syndrome (PCOS) battle. However, inactive pregnant women who eat lots of sugar and processed foods can find themselves in the same boat. Doctors and experts compound the problem by advising pregnant women to favor carbohydrates, usually as a way to combat morning sickness in the first trimester. This, along with the poor quality of most of our calcium- and iron-rich animal foods, sets a woman up for hormonal imbalances that could last through her pregnancy.

In order to lower androgens, strive to keep insulin low and avoid factory-farmed dairy and beef. And don't use pregnancy as an excuse to overindulge.

Light Hairs

Thyroxine, another pregnancy hormone, may promote fine, unpigmented hair—like the peachy fuzz on a cute little chick. It's not nearly as bothersome as the thicker, dark hair caused by testosterone. At least it wasn't for me. Because of PCOS, I had struggled with dark hair growth most of my adult life. But once the condition was gone, thanks to the Primal diet, light hair replaced dark during my second pregnancy.

Skin Changes

Some pregnancy hormones actually improve the skin, and some don't do it any good at all. Aim to keep the following hormones in perfect balance and you can enjoy the benefits of pregnancy.

- **Progesterone**—The hormone responsible for maintaining pregnancy in the first trimester acts as a relaxant on our muscles and brains, which is why pregnant women feel slower, weaker, sleepier, and sadder. But in the right amounts, it can also produce a more youthful, wrinkle-free appearance.

- **Estradiol**—You could call this hormone anti-progesterone: It's a stimulant, promoting mental clarity, alertness, and a pregnant woman's enhanced sense of smell. If it weren't for estradiol, pregnancy would be a real downer. In fact, when it's in proper balance, your nine months can be downright exhilarating. Estradiol improves blood flow to the skin, increases the water content, minimizing the appearance of fine lines, and helps to slough off old cells—all of which adds up to smoother, more beautiful skin. If it is opposed by too much testosterone, however, it can cause clogged pores.

- **Testosterone**—This is the naughty hormone responsible for unwanted hair growth and acne. That's because it rises slightly during pregnancy, causing an increase in sebum (oil) production.

- **Relaxin**—This makes labor possible by loosening the joints in preparation for delivery. However, there are negative side effects: weakened collagen, which makes you more susceptible to wrinkles and stretch marks. But if your hormones are in balance, progesterone will work to soften skin.

- **Insulin**—The hormone that contributes to belly fat also contributes to the growth of capillaries, which we know can lead to spider veins. Insulin is thought to be an adaptive hormone, allowing mother and baby to store more fat in the third trimester. But if too much of it is circulating in the blood, the ovaries will become over-stimulated and produce excess androgens (male hormones). The result? Unwanted hair growth, acne, and head hair loss.

Melanocyte-Stimulating Hormone (MSH)—MSH is a pituitary hormone that stimulates the production of pigment, making us more susceptible to sun damage.

Acne

Acne is probably the most embarrassing and noticeable skin change that can take place during pregnancy. It's most common in the first trimester, before estradiol production surpasses testosterone production. The following are steps you can take to combat acne during pregnancy:

* **Dairy**—Hypersensitivity to the hormones in dairy fat is not uncommon. If you have increased your dairy consumption to boost your Vitamin A, K2, and calcium, that might be the cause of acne. Cut it out of your diet for a few days to see if anything changes. You might be able to add dairy back after the estradiol kicks in in the second trimester (you should be okay with butter, or at least ghee, even before that).

* **Insulin**—If you are eating a high carb diet—due to a meat aversion, cravings, addictions, or whatever—your insulin will probably be higher than normal, causing excess testosterone. Go easy on the carbs and try to buffer them with fat and protein at every snack and meal.

* **Allergies**—Pregnant women have somewhat lowered immune systems. This mechanism protects the fetus from being rejected by the body, but it can also result in greater sensitivity to food. Allergies can provoke inflammation and a cascade of acne-causing hormones. If you find that you are more sensitive to foods while pregnant, you should be very strict with avoiding sugar and include plenty of anti-inflammatory foods like spinach, oranges, and cod liver oil.

* **Magnesium**—Boosting magnesium can help with acne. The calcium from dairy can lead to low magnesium levels, even if you take a supplement. So, again, try eliminating dairy, eating plenty of fresh vegetables, and supplementing your diet with magnesium (if you aren't already).

Acne *is* controllable with diet and lifestyle changes, but it can take time to identify the cause. If modifying your diet doesn't resolve the problem immediately, here are a few topical products that can help:

* **Witch Hazel**—This natural anti-inflammatory has been used topically for centuries. It won't cure the acne, but it may help to reduce its appearance.

* **Alpha Hydroxy and Glycolic Acids**—These acids are derived from fruits and can be used at home to promote faster skin cell turnover.

* **Blue Light Therapy**—Exposure to blue spectrum light helps kill bacteria below the surface, reducing breakouts and preventing them temporar-

ily. Many spas offer this, but it can get expensive; you need to do it a few times a week.

* **Tea Tree Oil**—An essential oil used topically to kill bacteria. It's less drying than benzoyl peroxide and can help reduce the length and severity of breakouts.

Darkening Skin

Melasma or Cloasma—"the mask of pregnancy"—is the darker skin color some women get; it usually affects the nose, forehead, and cheeks. Estradiol and MSH cause the production of more melanin during pregnancy, which is the name for the skin's pigment. This, coupled with the effects of the sun, can cause a darkening effect on the face. It's not serious and will fade after delivery. It helps to keep your face out of the sun, and some women have luck with natural remedies like topical Vitamin C products and alpha hydroxyl acids; both can lighten and exfoliate the skin.

Other parts of your body can darken during pregnancy, too: The areolas, genitals, moles, freckles, the palms of the hands, and the linea nigra (the line descending from the navel to the pubic bone). These changes have nothing to do with the sun and everything to do with the rise of MSH, which increases melanocytes. Researchers are not entirely sure why.

Wound Healing and Cesarean Scars

Following a Primal diet and lifestyle will not only keep you in optimum health during pregnancy, it can help you to avoid invasive labor. (Except perhaps for women who lack the ideal skeleton for childbirth; adult bones are one thing diet and lifestyle changes can't fix.) In America, long labors often lead to a Cesarean section. If your blood sugar is low, for example, or if you are afraid or stressed out during labor, you risk a Cesarean since both conditions inhibit the release of oxytocin, the hormone responsible for labor contractions. If it is low, labor may not progress. When it does not progress, doctors typically look for ways to speed it up.

Cesarean section is an invasive practice that, most of the time, is totally unnecessary. I don't want to diminish their horror; I know how bad it feels to see a great labor get manipulated into a bad labor, with the accompanying fear, the glucose IV drips, and the drugs. But if it happens, it's not the end of the world. The important thing is that you have a beautiful new baby! Rejoice in that. You'll be left with a scar, but the healing of that you *can* control.

Most doctors today make their incisions low and horizontal, so scars aren't visible when you wear a bathing suit. But no matter where your incision is made, take the necessary care of your scar so it heals well. Like just about everything else to do with your body, how fast and how well your scar heals has everything to do with inner health.

Phases of Wound Healing

There are three phases of wound healing. The first, which lasts up to five days, is the inflammatory stage. This is when white blood cells rush to keep the wound clean and free of infectious bacteria.

Stage two, the proliferative phase, lasts a few weeks. This is when hormone balance and good nutrition are imperative. Fibroblasts—the skin cells we learned about in chapter 7—migrate to the wound to suture it together with new collagen. Keeping the wound warm and moist with healing herb compresses—a method used for tens of thousands of years—helps facilitate this process. These days we generally ingest our herbs, but there is still a benefit to using moist topical applications.

The final, remodeling phase can last for up to two years. You will be building new collagen the whole time so be sure to keep nutrition optimal. While you no longer need to use herbal compresses and moist towels, there is one topical application that might be useful: silicone sheets. There is no conclusive evidence for why these work, but they do reduce the appearance of scars.

Herbs and Supplements for Wound Healing

+ **Zinc**—An all-around wound healer that, if taken up to six weeks before surgery, has been shown to dramatically speed up recovery and reduce scarring. For specific foods containing zinc, refer to chapter 12.

+ **Vitamin C**—Another important nutrient for wound healing. If you've been following this book, you are probably loading up on Vitamin C to prevent stretch marks. But it's especially important in postoperative patients because surgery can deplete Vitamin C. Ideal intake after surgery is 1 gram per day or more. Supplements are helpful, but it is easily obtained from Vitamin C-rich foods (including citrus, red peppers, rose hip tea, berries, and many other fruits and vegetables).

+ **Bromelain**—A powerful anti-inflammatory that provides some pain relief in addition to wound healing. I always use bromelain after injuring myself.

- **Comfrey**—A natural skin-healing herb that you can take fresh or powdered. Comfrey encourages the regrowth of skin cells and is ideal as a compress. Fresh macerated leaves or powdered root made into a paste with water can be applied to the incision and covered with a bandage. The wound will absorb some of the comfrey so apply more periodically. Leave this bandage on until the incision has closed.

- **Chlorella**—A popular super food that has been shown to speed up wound healing by promoting new cell growth, it can be taken internally or used in a compress.

- **Sunlight**—Patients who are exposed to sunlight (not directly on the wound, however) exhibit faster healing, no doubt thanks to the Vitamin D.

- **Gotu Kola**—Used in Asia for centuries, Gotu Kola can help remove scar tissue, particularly keloid scars; they might even prevent scars when applied topically. Gotu Kola is often taken internally but not if you are pregnant. In that case, apply a compress soaked in tea made from the dried herb.

- **Aloe**—This succulent plant has been used throughout history for healing wounds and minimizing scars. Aloe taken directly from the plant is best. It can be used either on a fresh wound or a healing scar.

- **Calendula**—An orange-colored flower that can be applied as a tea or salve to help remove scar tissue after it has already formed. It can also be used to heal wounds and minimize scarring.

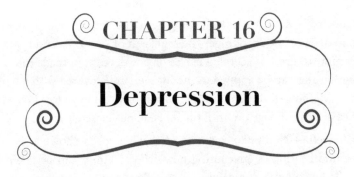

CHAPTER 16

Depression

Depression Isn't Attractive

Our moods affect our physical appearance in some pretty noticeable ways. We don't care how we look. We eat badly and don't take care of ourselves. Our posture slumps. We smoke and drink more. We have no drive or motivation to exercise. We don't smile as much. It leaves us feeling and looking dull and ugly.

Depression is related to all of the physical imperfections we've been learning how to prevent. For example, the rise in cortisol that accompanies some types of depression can lead to weight gain and premature aging. And magnesium deficiency, which also contributes to depression, can lead to bone problems and hunched posture.

Depression can happen any time in a person's life, but it is particularly common in pregnant and postpartum women because of the dramatic hormonal changes that take place.

Antenatal Depression

Most of the time, increased estradiol elevates the moods of pregnant women, but 20 percent experience depression anyway. That isn't surprising given how common hormonal imbalances are. But pregnancy *should* be a time of elation, not sadness and frustration.

Of course, every pregnant woman is likely to experience *some* mood swings, particularly in the first trimester when the body is still adjusting to the rise in hormones. There is a difference, however, between fleeting feelings of sadness and depression. Mood swings are an emotional rollercoaster that can be disruptive. Depression cuts much deeper; it's an emotional fog that never lifts, destructive to the victim and everyone around her. Worse, depression affects the fetus. If a mother isn't sleeping or has lost her appetite, or, conversely, if she is overeating and sleeping too much, brain development is compromised.

Research suggests that depression during pregnancy contributes to premature delivery, low birth weight, and preeclampsia. It has also been associated with smaller head circumference, increased risk of surgical delivery interventions, lower APGAR scores, and infants who cry more often and have irregular sleep patterns.

If a woman suffers from depression, she must take steps to resolve hormonal imbalances, in addition to any contributing social circumstances (more on that in chapter 17).

Baby Blues

Natal-related depression comes in a few different forms, ranging from mild to severe, visiting a woman throughout her pregnancy or after. You have likely heard of postpartum depression but there are milder forms as well, lasting anywhere from a few days to a few weeks. Up to 70 percent of all women experience some form of postpartum blues. The two less extreme forms are:

Delivery Blues—As a result of sudden reductions in progesterone and estradiol, postpartum women can experience a brief overwhelming sadness. This usually resolves within three days after delivery. Not all women experience this, so dramatic hormone dips after delivery may not be the cause of delivery blues.

Baby Blues—This is definitely hormone-related. It lasts a little longer than delivery blues, but resolves within a couple of weeks. Again, not all women experience this.

Thankfully, these depressive symptoms do not last and are not considered serious. Nevertheless, they do dampen what should be a miraculous and joyous experience.

Postpartum Depression

When depression is more than fleeting and causes a detachment from the baby, it is referred to as postpartum depression (PPD). PPD can sometimes be related to bitter circumstance, but it is generally caused by hormonal and biochemical imbalances which are themselves brought on by nutrient deficiencies, low-fat diets, excess sugar, and exposure to stress and environmental estrogens. Around 12-16 percent of women experience full-blown PPD.

Symptoms of Postpartum Depression

Women suffering from PPD are not as responsive to infant cues. More seriously, they may have negative, even violent, thoughts about their babies. Such behavior can lead to extreme feelings of guilt: A mother expects to love her child intensely. Generally these women will exhibit overwhelming fatigue and some kind of appetite disturbance—either overeating or undereating.

Symptoms will usually resolve on their own within, on average, seven months, but they can sometimes last well over a year. A woman who suspects she has PPD should be screened for anemia and thyroid disease as they are often implicated. The effects PPD have on a baby can be profound and should not be underestimated.

How Depression Hurts the Baby

Babies need stimulation to form neural connections; it is essential to the development of their brains. Depressed women suffering from fatigue and apathy will not want to spend quality time with their babies. Studies have shown that infants of depressed mothers have higher levels of the stress hormones that inhibit brain development. Furthermore, they are more likely to display violent or dysfunctional behavior when they enter school.

Research has exhibited other risks: poor mother-infant attachment, delayed cognitive and linguistic skills, impaired emotional development, and behavioral issues. One study showed that these developmental delays remain even if the mother is treated four months after delivery.

Postpartum Psychosis

Postpartum psychosis is incredibly rare, affecting only 1 in 500-1,000 new mothers. It is entirely different from PPD. Andrea Yates, the woman who drowned her five children in the bathtub, had postpartum psychosis *not* PPD. The onset of this condition is severe and quick, and personality changes are truly beyond the person's control; they have lost touch with reality. Family members or friends who see signs of postpartum psychosis should consider it a medical emergency and respond appropriately.

Symptoms of Postpartum Psychosis

- Severe depression
- Unwillingness to eat or sleep
- Frantic energy
- Delusions or false beliefs
- Hallucinations (hearing voices or seeing things that are not real)
- Thoughts of harming or killing the baby

Anxiety

In the pregnant woman, different hormones can contribute to and even prevent anxiety. Whether the mother experiences anxiety depends on the levels of these hormones. An imbalance of estradiol can contribute to anxiety since it is stimulating to the brain. Estradiol makes the nerves in the frontal lobe more excitable. Overly excited nerves in this region of the brain can cause anxiety.

The stimulating effect of estradiol offers an evolutionary advantage. A woman who is on heightened alert for danger during pregnancy and after delivery can be a better protector. But a woman who is overstimulated as a result of too much estradiol can become anxious and incapacitated. Even the smallest details of life seem overwhelming. At this point in history, when the daily life-threatening dangers our ancestors faced are gone, severe anxiety is not only a disadvantage, it is a sign of ill health.

I experienced full-blown non-pregnancy-related anxiety just a few years ago. I was in a serious mountain biking accident just days after a terrible family tragedy. I flew off my bike, which was going about 20 miles per hour, and hit the ground with my chin. I fell unconscious and was found later that morning by a couple of women who were out for a hike; miraculously, they were nurses. I don't remember any of this, but apparently they woke me up, gave me water, and helped get me to a hospital. My first memory was later that evening when the doctor scraped the rocks out of my wounds and stitched up my chin. The next few days are a blur, and it was months before I could retain short-term or recover long-term memories. In addition to confusion, I also developed anxiety. The flood of fight-or-flight hormones like cortisol and adrenaline took a long time to balance and I often felt out of control and unsafe; I had severe, heart-pounding anxiety attacks. At times I feared I was going to die, and I worried I might be suffering long-term brain damage. And then I remembered something: In all of the confusion and helplessness of recovery somehow sugar had been re-introduced into my diet. Maybe that was slowing my recovery! I had been eating sugar again for just a few months but with the hormonal imbalances that ensued after the trauma, three months was long enough to have such a strong effect. I quickly eliminated sugar and was more careful about what I ate in general, and within days I was feeling less fearful. Within a couple of weeks, I had my last anxiety attack.

The reason why anxiety hit me so hard was because my stress hormones were already elevated. When a person eats a sugary food, the body responds by secreting insulin to lower the blood's sugar level. This is fine when we eat a reasonable amount of carbohydrates and commit to low glycemic meals. But when we eat a lot of sugar, our bodies respond with a surge of insulin to lower the sugar in the blood. When this happens, another hormone must counter that action. Not only does cortisol help to keep your blood sugar levels even, it prepares the body for fight or flight by turning on the sympathetic nervous system, which raises our heart rate, making us highly sensitive, wakeful, and prepared for action (as opposed to the parasympathetic nervous system, which helps us rest, digest, and deliver babies). This is great when we're in danger, but can be very confusing and scary when we're sitting quietly at home.

If I hadn't had the bicycle accident, my stress response hormones wouldn't have risen so dramatically and neither would my vulnerability to the effects of sugar. Likewise, if a pregnant woman were not already burdened with extra cortisol she could better handle anxiety. Pregnancy itself does not cause anxiety but it does predispose us if we exacerbate the situation with bad food choices and additional stressors. Our bodies, if treated well, are well-equipped to find equilibrium.

Take great care to avoid anxiety during pregnancy. It is harmful to you and your fetus. One study found that children of anxious mothers were more likely to develop attention deficit/hyperactivity disorder, or ADHD. One possible reason for this is that cortisol crosses the placenta and can disturb the developmental process.

In addition to elevated cortisol, anxiety can be caused by a drop in progesterone. This usually happens postpartum but it can occur any time during the nine months of pregnancy and can be a sign of preterm labor. Studies have confirmed a link between anxiety and miscarriage, anxiety and preterm birth, and anxiety and preeclampsia. This is probably because they are all related to a drop in progesterone.

Causes of Depression

The Role of Pregnancy Hormones in Depression

The chemical changes that take place in a pregnant woman are profound and dramatic. Hormones of all types flood her body and then suddenly plummet after delivery. Both scenarios are kindling for mood disorders. Every pregnant and postpartum woman experiences the rise and fall of these hormones. Ideally, the negative, mood-lowering impact of one will be offset by another.

- **Estradiol** boosts the production of the neurotransmitters serotonin, norepinephrine, and dopamine. For most pregnant women this is a positive. However, estradiol plummets suddenly and dramatically after pregnancy and can cause a type of withdrawal or, if the woman was feeling low before pregnancy, simply bring her back down to that state.

- **Progesterone** generally has a positive, calming effect on pregnant women. However, the withdrawal after delivery can be dramatic.

- **Corticotropin-releasing Hormone (CRH) and Adrenocorticotropic Hormone (ACTH)** signal the adrenal glands to produce stress hormones such as cortisol.

- **Cortisol** levels automatically drop after delivery, unless the woman is depressed.

- **Prolactin** is produced during lactation and can cause a dip in dopamine—a neurotransmitter responsible for the feeling of pleasure, motivation, and attention. During pregnancy this is offset by estradiol. During breastfeeding it is offset by oxytocin. If a woman does not breastfeed, there is no protection against the dip in dopamine. Without breastfeeding, prolactin levels will return to normal within three months.

- **Thyroxine** is a thyroid hormone that, when low, can cause symptoms of depression. Thyroxine may dip after delivery.

Neurotransmitters

The other set of chemicals that may be responsible for some level of the blues are the neurotransmitters serotonin, dopamine, and norepinephrine. To understand a neurotransmitter's role in depression, let's take a closer look at what is happening inside the brain.

Chemical messages—i.e., all communication with the brain and the body such as emotions, behavior, temperature, appetite, and many other functions—pass through the brain beginning as an electrical impulse. This electrical impulse is picked up by the neuron and quickly changed to a chemical impulse or neurotransmitter. The neurotransmitters actually carry the messages from neuron to neuron via the synapse, which is kind of like a little bridge between neurons. Once they reach their destination and deliver their message, they return to the sending neuron where they are reabsorbed (called reuptake) and are ready to be reused.

The neurotransmitters serotonin, dopamine, and norepinephrine regulate messages of emotion, sexuality, sleep, and reactions to stress. It is thought that low levels of these neurotransmitters contribute to depression. When there is not enough serotonin, for example, it will not make its way back to the sending neuron and undergo the process of reuptake. Now the sending neuron will be incapable of releasing another message with serotonin. If there are no messages sent, no messages will be received, leading to symptoms of depression.

Dr. Julia Sacher and her team of researchers found in a recent study that levels of the enzyme monoamine oxidase A (MAO-A) increase in the female brain in proportion to the drop in estrogen immediately after delivery. This enzyme can break down the neurotransmitters serotonin, dopamine, and norepinephrine, leading to a deficit.

Nutrient Deficiencies

Hormone balance and a healthy level of neurotransmitters cannot be achieved without nutrients—something most of us don't realize as we stuff our faces with meal after meal of nutrient-deficient foods. It is imperative that pregnant and lactating women think carefully about what they put into their bodies. Researchers in Canada reported that the "depletion of nutrient reserves throughout pregnancy can increase a woman's risk for maternal depression."

Depression has been shown to correlate with low levels of magnesium, selenium, folate, Vitamin B12, calcium, and iron. And the neurotransmitters serotonin, norepinephrine, and dopamine all require a steady supply of tryptophan, Vitamin B6, and tyrosine.

The process that the body must go through to make neurotransmitters is complicated. You don't just eat them in food and you can't take them as a tablet because they don't cross the blood brain barrier. The body must have enough iron and Vitamin B3 to convert tryptophan into a compound known as 5-hydroxy-L-tryptophan (5-HTP). But that's not enough. It must also convert 5-HTP into its usable form, pyridoxyl-5-phosphate (P5P). Without enough 5-HTP and P5P (and therefore enough of the specific vitamin and mineral precursors to synthesize them), the brain will be lacking in neurotransmitters and depression will result.

Parental Investment

There may also be an evolutionary link to postpartum depression. When a woman's situation is such that she has suffered some kind of familial misfortune, her brain may kick in to an evolutionary mode known as survival of the species.

In nature, animals are able to recognize inopportune times for rearing their young. In times of scarcity, for instance, they know they will be more successful in passing on their genes if they abandon their young and try again when conditions improve. Researchers hypothesize a similar, perhaps even more sensitive, evolutionary mechanism in humans. It makes sense since human parents must "invest" many more years and much more effort into raising their young. This investment is unmatched in any other species.

Human babies are 100 percent dependent upon their parents for their first few years. They require constant care and supervision. Since we must invest so much time and energy into raising a single child, the conditions had better be favorable for success. Researchers suggest that nature might be influencing a woman to distance herself from her infant if conditions for a positive outcome are unfavorable; this can present as depression. The distancing can happen when there is not enough food to feed the mother and the baby, when the infant does not appear to be developing well or has some major health problem, and when the mother does not have sufficient support systems—either social or nutritional, or both.

You would think this evolutionary mechanism would have dropped off as life got easier. But evolution doesn't happen that fast. Although we often think of ourselves as "above animals" we still have the same thousands of years of programming.

Bottle Feeding and Child Loss

Another evolutionary mechanism at work is our body's ability to detect and respond to changes in our hormones after pregnancy. If a woman opts not to breastfeed and the hormonal processes caused by lactation come to a halt, the body recognizes three possible causes: miscarriage, loss, or death of the child. Research suggests that postpartum depression can be caused by the *perceived* loss of a child, triggering profound grief and depression in the mother.

In the paper *Bottle Feeding Simulates Child Loss: Postpartum Depression and Evolutionary Medicine*, the authors examined "the decision people make to unwittingly depart from one of the defining features of mammalian evolution: to bottle feed rather than breastfeed their infants." They noted that prior to the last hundred years—before plastic bottles, rubber nipples, and formula—a mother had only one option for feeding infants: her breasts. "For 99.9 percent of human evolutionary history the decision not to breastfeed would have been tantamount to committing infanticide."

How much does a woman's mind control this evolutionary response to lowered prolactin? Researchers don't know. Clearly every woman who opts to use a bottle is not miserably depressed, so some of us do overcome these evolutionary cues. But women who are at high risk for depression, who don't have great nutrition or support systems, or who have low neurotransmitters might want to consider breastfeeding.

Conquering Depression

Depression can be overcome naturally. A woman should take responsibility for her health, no matter how challenging this can be in times of stress and depression. Regular exercise, a Primal-style diet, and social support should be enough to overcome and prevent most pregnancy-caused depressions. Higher-risk women should think about herbs and supplements.

Herbs and Supplements

You can seek mental help and exercise but if you don't eat well, your efforts will likely fail. Years of ill treatment to the brain and body can require years of recovery. There are many supplements that can help speed the process. If you are pregnant or breastfeeding, speak with your doctor regarding the safety of the following:

- **SAM-e (S-adenosylmethionine)** helps the brain produce neurotransmitters. People with depression are often low on SAM-e and supplements have shown to be effective. SAM-e should be avoided by people with bipolar disorder as it can cause manic episodes.

- **Amino acids** tryptophan and tyrosine can help boost the neurotransmitters serotonin, norepinephrine, and dopamine.

- **Zinc** supplementation has been shown to ameliorate depressive symptoms (men and women suffering from depression have been shown to have low zinc levels, with the lowest levels found in the most depressed).

- **St. John's Wort** is probably the most popular herbal anti-depressant on the market. It is used to treat depression, anxiety, and sleep disorders. The active ingredients are thought to boost serotonin levels. Research has shown that it is effective with milder depressions but not severe depression. The safety of the herb in nursing mothers is unknown.

- **Gingko Biloba**, which comes from the leaves of one of the earth's oldest trees, helps to improve mental clarity, alertness, and memory, and can be helpful in those with mild depression.

- **Kava** has been approved for use to relieve symptoms of anxiety, insomnia, and depression in Europe. There have been reports of liver problems associated with taking kava but there is no concrete evidence.

- **Passion Flower** can be used as a sedative and to help with insomnia; it can also relieve anxiety and nervousness.

Exercise

Exercise should be done regularly. Here are the best activities for balancing hormones:

- **Weight bearing exercise and moderate aerobics**—Not doing these actually disturbs hormone balance.

- **Yoga**—Studies have shown that it reduces stress hormones by up to 80 percent after just 30 minutes. Done regularly, this can boost positive hormonal shifts.

- **Meditation**—Relaxation and controlled breathing lowers stress hormones naturally.

Social Support

Psychological disorders are often exacerbated by a weak support system. This is not an easy problem to fix, but if emotional disorders are an issue, the sooner they are resolved the better. Women who experience psychological distress during pregnancy will likely suffer from it after the baby is born. As important as a good diet is to our health, so is getting support and love from those closest to you. If fighting or spousal abuse are a problem, seek counseling and, if necessary, leave the situation. Keeping a healthy support system might take some effort, but it is critical to the health of the baby. If you are feeling lonely, look into joining a meetup.com group, which links people with similar interests.

Alternative Treatments

Acupuncture, chiropractic, and applied Kinesiology may offer relief for depression. They can also positively affect your hormone balance. See chapter 17 for more information.

Side Effects of SSRIs

In the brain, neurons send messages of all kinds, including those of well-being. They do this by sending chemicals like serotonin from one presynaptic neuron through the synapse to another postsynaptic neuron. In people who are depressed serotonin doesn't always make it past the synapse and into the postsynaptic neuron. Instead they are either destroyed by monoamine oxidase (MAO) or reabsorbed by the presynaptic neuron. In either case, the message does not get sent and the person does not feel good. SSRIs, or selective serotonin reuptake inhibitors, include Fluoxetine anti-depressants (tradenames include Zoloft, Prozac, Paxil, and Lexapro). These drugs prevent the presynaptic reuptake of serotonin, which may allow more serotonin to be absorbed by the postsynaptic receptor, thus successfully sending messages of well-being.

SSRIs do *not* actually help the brain to create more serotonin (only good nutrition and low stress can do that), but they do help the brain to better use what supply it has. This might sound great at first but drugs don't come without side effects. Some of the most commonly troublesome effects of SSRIs are sleep disturbances, sexual dysfunction, and weight gain. A recent study funded by Kaiser Permanente found a correlation between SSRIs and autism. Most of the cases were in babies whose mothers took them during the first trimester. Additionally, I think it is important to consider the fact that these drugs are quite new, relatively speaking, and their potential complications may not be revealed for years to come. Furthermore, it is not even possible to test the side effects that drug interactions may produce. There are literally thousands of possible combinations of prescription medication. The effect one has on the body in the presence of another is mostly unknown.

Other studies have shown that, in some infants, Fluoxetine is associated with colic and behavioral disorders. It would hardly be surprising if SSRIs negatively impact the growing fetus and infant. In fact, a meta-analysis, including nine studies, showed an increased risk of premature birth and low birth weight when SSRIs are taken in the third trimester.

Probably the most serious side effect of SSRIs is serotonin syndrome (SS). This is usually caused by mixing an SSRI—either in the beginning of use or at an increase of dosage—with other drugs, including opioids, cocaine, Ritalin, and ecstasy. The symptoms of SS include agitation, restlessness, rapid heartbeat, hallucinations, increased body temperature, loss of coordination, diarrhea, vomiting. The condition can be deadly.

Due to the side effects of SSRIs, the limited evidence of the actual efficacy, and the lack of long-term, unbiased research, psychotropic drugs should be avoided, especially by pregnant and nursing women. This doesn't mean that pregnant and nursing mothers should have to suffer, however. Serotonin production can be enhanced quite easily, as we will see in the next chapter.

Fructose Malabsorption

Chances are if you have an intolerance to fructose, called fructose malabsorption, you've had it all your life and didn't just develop it in pregnancy. I'm mentioning it here because it's relatively unknown and can be a big factor in female depression.

Researchers from the University of Innsbruck in Austria found a high correlation between women with fructose malabsorption and depression (they did not find the same in men). Another Spanish study found that 71 percent of the depressed adolescents studied had sugar intolerance, compared with 15 percent of controls. This is a huge margin and the possibility of a depressed woman having fructose malabsorption should not be overlooked.

The test for fructose malabsorption is the same simple breath test used to determine lactose intolerance. In fact, getting a test for both is a good idea; studies have shown that an even greater instance of depression can result when these disorders are combined. Dr. Emily Deans, an MD with interests in evolutionary psychiatry, clarified the cause of the connection between women, fructose malabsorption, and depression on her blog. Why is the connection specifically with women and not men? The answer, she says, is because men have more tryptophan than women.

"Fructose (and lactose) can react chemically with tryptophan, the amino acid precursor for our important happy chemical, serotonin. The sugars can degrade tryptophan so that there isn't as much available to be absorbed into the body. And, indeed, fructose malabsorbers have lower levels of tryptophan in the serum than normal controls."

She goes on to question why the symptoms of depression would be confined to women, and concludes that "estrogen made the big difference. Estrogen activates an enzyme called hepatic tryptophan 2,3 dioxygenase that shifts the metabolism of tryptophan from making serotonin (happy) to making kynurenic (not happy). Women already have lower serum levels of tryptophan than men do (which may be part of the reason why we are more vulnerable to depression in the first place), so screwing up whatever available tryptophan in the diet with fructose may lead to even lower levels, and thus depression."

I have fructose malabsorbption and, while I didn't know about the disorder until I ran into Dr. Deans' articles, I basically figured it out myself years before. I had noticed that fruit caused extreme sadness, acne, and candida (due to the fermentation of the unabsorbed sugars). Controlling FM is a little more complicated than simply eliminating fruit so I would suggest that anyone who suspects they might have this condition get tested. Then learn about the foods that can be problematic, like onions and garlic.

CHAPTER 17

Strategies and Supplements For Hormone Balance

The diet outlined in this book may help a woman balance her hormones rather quickly. Healing may prove elusive, however, if certain nutrients are low, if inflammation and stress are high, or if activity levels are too low (or sometimes too high, what we call over-exercising)—and that's even if you are eating some version of a Paleo or Primal diet. A healing, hormone-balancing diet—just like the diet to rebuild connective tissue—should focus on anti-inflammatory foods, protein, healthy fats, and nutrients from a variety of organs and plant foods.

Hormone Disruptors

Xenoestrogens

Pollution, exposure to plastics, chemicals, and conventional beef treated with synthetic hormones can contribute to hormonal imbalances because they contain xenoestrogens (synthetic, or environmental estrogens). These environmental estrogens wreak havoc on our delicate hormonal processes by tricking the body into thinking that there is too much estrogen, causing it to produce excessive amounts of other hormones in an effort to balance everything out.

Excess Insulin

To improve insulin sensitivity, you need to restrict carbs, particularly sugar. By this I do not mean *eliminate* carbs; that can lead to excess cortisol. When blood sugar levels are low, the body responds by secreting cortisol in order to boost the blood's level of sugar. A person needs to be very careful to keep their blood sugar even and their stress levels reduced when they are on a low-carb diet. An easier strategy is to eat carbohydrates, but limit them to around 100 grams if you aren't pregnant or breastfeeding, and a little more if you are. As with any dietary advice, however, keep in mind that we are all different and our needs vary.

Specific Nutrients and Supplements

The following nutrients have been found to be particularly useful for balancing hormones and managing depression.

* **Cholesterol** is very important for the brain. Scientists have effectively turned Americans against dietary cholesterol while pushing dangerous cholesterol-lowering statin drugs. This is a mistake. Low levels of cholesterol can lead to depression, anxiety, and impulsive, violent behavior, and research has shown that low serum cholesterol is not safe. What is safe is focusing on making sound dietary choices in line with ancient traditions. Molecular biologist Amitabha Chattopadhyay and his team of researchers have shown that long-term use of statin drugs caused significant change in the structure and function of serotonin cell receptors. Foods that are high in cholesterol, like liver and egg yolk, are healthy and should not be restricted.

* **Cod liver oil** contains DHA that has been shown in countless studies to reduce depressive symptoms. Additionally, we need a healthy balance of omega-3 to omega-6 fatty acids to maintain balanced hormones and cod liver oil offers the omega-3 lacking in the average American diet. A pregnant woman should be taking between 2-4 teaspoons for DHA and Vitamins A and D.

* **Chromium** can improve insulin resistance, hence balancing the hormonal cascade resulting from high blood sugar. It can also help a woman reduce cravings for "comfort foods." Though the supplement has not been studied in pregnant women, it has no established risks and is considered safe.

* **Bioidentical progesterone** might be useful for women experiencing anxiety during pregnancy. It can also be helpful for women with estrogen dominance which, these days, is most of us. There are no contraindications for pregnant women; just be sure to consult your doctor. If you don't need progesterone, you shouldn't be taking it.

* **Selenium** was shown in a recent study to alleviate depressive symptoms in pregnant women taking 100 mcg daily throughout pregnancy. Brazil

nuts have the highest selenium content of any food, at 70-90 mcg per nut. Next in line are cod, tuna, rice, and halibut.

* **Vitamin C** can enhance hormone balance. This very accessible vitamin is involved in almost every biochemical process in the human body. It plays an important role in the manufacturing of hormones.

* **B Vitamins** such as B12, B6, and folate are all important for female hormone balance. Sources of B6 include meats, nuts, and vegetables. Folate mainly comes from vegetables and B12 comes only from animal sources.

* **Magnesium** deficiency is common in just about everyone and plays a big role in depression and hormone balance. Vegetables and nuts are good sources and magnesium supplements have been shown to be highly effective.

* **Saw Palmetto** is an herb that can be used after the baby is born. It may help lower the androgens responsible for the dark hair growth and head hair loss common in PCOS sufferers. Saw palmetto is thought to reduce levels of 5-alpha reductase—an enzyme responsible for converting testosterone into the stronger androgen dihydrotestosterone. High concentrations of dihydrotestosterone are implicated in benign prostatic hypertrophy and male pattern baldness, as well as female pattern baldness and hirsutism.

* **DIM** is available as a supplement and as a naturally occurring phytonutrient in cruciferous vegetables like broccoli and kale. DIM promotes beneficial estrogen metabolism, which can improve hormone balance.

Leaky Gut and the Paleo Elimination Diet

It isn't always easy to pinpoint specific imbalances or the cause of certain digestive problems. Our bodies require a wide spectrum of nutrients; if any of those drops too low, symptoms may result. If serious digestive illness or a lowered immune system is present, you may require additional supplements or an elimination diet to achieve a healthy hormone balance.

When gut health is compromised, a person can seem to be allergic to *everything*. While the reactions aren't really allergic, it may appear that way. Because so many things are possible causes of digestive distress—carbohydrate malabsorption issues, leaky gut, insufficient stomach acid or bile, inflammatory bowel conditions, low thyroid—it can be difficult to self-diagnose. Even doctors can miss the cause of the problems. If your digestion is gassy, if you have constipation or diarrhea, if your belly is distended, or if your stool is smelly, too frequent, or contains undigested food, you absolutely will not absorb all the nutrients you eat and need. In time, the situation could lead to damage and inflammation of the intestine walls, which is very serious.

Leaky Gut

A weak intestinal lining means the cells are damaged and food molecules and waste particles can escape into the bloodstream. This is called leaky gut. Some of the possible causes include:

- Street drugs
- Alcohol, including beer and wine
- Nicotine
- Antibiotics
- Fermentation of carbohydrates from malabsorption issues
- NSAIDS (aspirin, ibuprofen, acetaminophen)
- Birth control pills
- Sugar
- Nutrient deficiencies
- Parasites, bacteria, and yeasts
- Inflammatory intestinal diseases (Chron's, celiac, colitis)
- Food allergies
- Stress

The intestines were designed to keep food perfectly contained for processing. Food needs to be completely broken down before it is safe to go traveling through the blood stream. Think of injecting a chewed up salad via a large needle. The salad is perfectly healthy but the body wouldn't see it that way. It would reject all of the foreign particles circulating through the blood—particles which are both unusable and highly toxic in that undigested form.

So when substances that are not completely broken down go circulating through the blood stream, the immune system will do everything it can to clean up the mess. This is when things get uncomfortable. Every time you eat, your immune system, which has a lot of jobs to do all day long, is stuck doing just one job—cleaning up a mess that shouldn't be there in the first place. A person can experience all sorts of pain and discomfort from this process.

Some symptoms of leaky gut can mimic allergic symptoms even when no allergies appear on an allergy test. Symptoms include:

+ Headaches
+ Joint pain
+ Rashes
+ Fatigue
+ Digestive problems
+ Fungal and yeast infections

The Paleo Elimination Diet

Healing from leaky gut and other digestive conditions isn't as easy as eliminating grains, legumes, PUFAs, sugar, and dairy. When the gut lining is seriously damaged, even vegetables and fruits can be harmful. The fructose in fruit can cause the sort of severe gas pains that accompany lactose intolerance. A simple cup of coffee can cause rashes and hyperactivity.

When this is the case, the best approach is often a meat-based elimination diet, as meat rarely causes reactions in most people. I personally designed this diet for myself and had amazing success with it. Due to the severe digestive problems I suffered as a result of celiac disease, I reacted to just about anything that grew in the ground. Lifelong neck and back pain vanished for the first time after I eliminated fruits and vegetables. In addition, my skin cleared up and I never saw another rash. My hormones had been balancing slowly on a regular Paleo diet for years but when I took it to this level, recovery was dramatic. I have seen this diet help many people and truly believe in its efficacy. There are many restrictions, which can be challenging. In addition, important nutrients will be missing from the diet so only do it for a month if your are not pregnant and no more than a week if you are. Throughout, be diligent about drinking kombucha for added B Vitamins and eating liver and other organs for magnesium, B Vitamins, Vitamin C (some of the many nutrients missing from muscle meats).

A meat-based elimination diet would begin with the following:

+ Raw or lightly cooked fresh meats and seafoods (not bacon and lunchmeats)
+ Sea salt
+ Organ meats
+ Chicken and fish bone broths

- Butter or ghee
- White rice for glucose (needed for fetal brain development and to maintain a healthy thyroid)
- Plain kombucha (this can be made at home—details are on my blog, ThePrimalParent.com—or purchased at a health food store)

After a week or two, slowly add foods back to determine specific sensitivities. The FODMAPs (Fermentable Oligo-, Di- and Mono-saccharides, and Polyols) from foods such as milk, fruit, onions, cabbage, and garlic, are commonly problematic in people with digestive problems.

The foods which are most nutritious and often the safest to start adding back include:

- Lemon or lime juice
- Olive and coconut oils
- Dark green leafy vegetables like spinach, kale, and chard

If these are well-tolerated, introduce one food back into the diet every day, beginning with eggs and non- FODMAP vegetables. Then move on to some of the more likely culprits, like fruit, dairy, spices, and other starches. Just be sure to add only one food per day at first; it can take many hours for symptoms to surface.

Sunshine

Vitamin D plays an important role in hormone balance and the sun is the best place to get it. The sun converts the cholesterol naturally present in our skin to the Vitamin D necessary for maintaining health on many levels. Vitamin D is important for regulating insulin secretion and balancing blood sugar, for improving thyroid function, for warding off depression and breast cancer, for maintaining calcium balance and strengthening bones, for killing bacteria, and for wound healing. Vitamin D isn't widely available through diet. It is found in the livers of animals, and these days we obtain synthetic variants in fortified milk. Our prime source of Vitamin D is through sun exposure. As I mentioned earlier, an hour or so per week in direct, overhead sunlight without sunscreen is enough to experience the many benefits of Vitamin D.

If you live in a northern climate, the weather might be too cold to lay out during the winter months. And in the spring, summer, and winter the sun is angled too low in the sky to effectively make the conversion of cholesterol to Vitamin D. (The conversion only happens when the solar UVB photons penetrate the skin at 290-315 nanometers. You can check the angle of the sun in your area each day on the US Naval Observatory website or with the iPhone app called D Minder.) When this is the case, you should supplement with cod liver oil.

Vitamin D is naturally occurring in cod liver oil, a supplement every pregnant and breastfeeding woman should be taking anyway. One teaspoon of regular cod liver oil offers 400-500 IU Vitamin D. According to the Weston A. Price Foundation, a pregnant or breastfeeding woman should take four teaspoons per day. Other adults should be taking two teaspoons per day.

The US RDA recommends 200 IU of Vitamin D per day but studies have concluded that this amount is insufficient. Reinhold Vieth, PhD, published a review of Vitamin D in the May 1999 *American Journal of Clinical Nutrition*; in it he reports that adults may need, at minimum, five times the RDA—or 1,000 IU daily—to derive health benefits. "Total-body sun exposure easily provides the equivalent of 250 µg (10000 IU) Vitamin D/d, suggesting that this is a physiologic limit."

Tanning Beds During the Winter Months

Another avenue for Vitamin D supplementation is tanning beds. Denver, albeit a sunny place, is so far north that the angle of the sun does not offer the right wavelength for the skin to convert cholesterol to Vitamin D during most of the year. It's too cold 7 or 8 months out of the year anyway. During the long winters here, I use a tanning bed once or twice a week to make up for the sunshine deficit.

You will want to choose a tanning bed which emits more UVB rays than UVA since UVB are the rays that cause the conversion from cholesterol to Vitamin D in our skin and UVAs are the rays which cause cancer. Many tanning beds are calibrated to emit up to 95 percent UVA rays. While these beds do tan the skin, they don't offer the benefit of Vitamin D and they can do long-term damage to the skin. Most salons, however, offer a scale of beds ranging from nearly 0 percent UVB to almost 100 percent UVB. Ask a salon technician for more information.

There have been no published studies to date indicating that tanning in a tanning bed is harmful to a fetus. The ultraviolet light exposure never reaches the baby. However, according to Dr. Joseph Mercola, the electromagnetic field

(EMFs), which are produced by the bed's magnetic ballasts, "are of major concern." Some newer beds use electronic ballasts that are thought to be safer.

The main concern for the baby is the risk of elevated body temperature. Pregnant women must take care not to let their body temperature exceed 102 degrees Fahrenheit. Hyperthermia can cause spinal malformations in developing fetuses. Of course, pregnant women will need to take the same care when laying out in direct sunlight.

The last concern with ultraviolet exposure is the effect it can have on the color of the skin. Pregnancy hormones make the skin more sensitive and prone to dark discoloration, or chloasma. Protecting the delicate skin on the face is advised, but keep the rest of your body unprotected or Vitamin D's much-needed benefits will be inhibited.

Alternative Therapies

Acupuncture

Acupuncture is an ancient Chinese healing modality that cures or manages conditions with the use of slender needles placed in very specific locations throughout the body. Acupuncture corrects the flow of energy, stimulating the body's ability to overcome illnesses or chronic conditions. It is used to correct everything from anxiety to depression to back pain and PMS.

In a 2004 study examining acupuncture's effect on insomnia, researchers reported that five weeks of acupuncture was associated with a significant increase of melatonin secretion. Subjects experienced relief of both their insomnia and anxiety, according to the study, which was published by the American Psychiatric Press.

Chiropractic

Chiropractic therapy uses adjustments to the spine to balance the overall health of the body's nervous system. These adjustments assist the body in establishing better coordination between the central and peripheral nervous systems. This coordination can help relieve everything from digestive problems to back pain and emotional problems.

PART IV

Loving Your New Body

A pregnant woman's body changes. There is no fighting the extra padding and larger belly and breasts. Most women experience some change in the texture or size of their breasts after they've stopped nursing. Some women find that they store fat in different places than they used to. Others may develop a small complication during a particularly stressful period in their pregnancy. These kinds of changes are to be expected and accepted.

There are also changes we don't expect, many of them beneficial, including a reduced breast cancer risk, better sex, and a greater acceptance of ourselves and our place in the world. Pregnancy changes our bodies and minds. To what degree we change is dependent upon our situation and the decisions we make before, during, and after pregnancy.

CHAPTER 18

Desirable Physical Effects of Pregnancy

There are other biped mammals on earth (the kangaroo, wallaby, spring-hare, kangaroo rat), but only humans walk with an alternating bipedal gait 100 percent of the time. (Giant Pangolins *can* walk with the alternating gait but they have four legs and are usually spotted walking on all fours.) Standing and walking upright have given human men and women an incredible evolutionary advantage; it's the posture that allowed us to make and use tools and to extract the most nutrient-dense substances from our surroundings. But it comes at a cost. According to Timothy Taylor, author of *The Prehistory of Sex*, "walking upright also means a modified pelvis that makes childbirth difficult and imposes a limit on fetal head size." Translation: Our birth canal narrowed. So while our incredibly efficient bodies excel at many things, childbirth is not one of them. It's not ideal for pregnancy either: Before making its way through an inadequately-sized canal, the fetus puts pressure on the mother's lungs, intestines, and ribs, among other things. It is no wonder that we are susceptible to a host of annoying conditions.

But let's look on the bright side, because there is one. Many of the changes caused by pregnancy turn into advantages—even rib expansion!

Strong Nails

We already know what pregnancy can do for your hair. Some women notice the same benefits to their nails: they get stronger and longer. This could be the result of hormones, but it could also be due to the pregnancy vitamins many women start taking when they find out they're pregnant.

Most women notice positive changes to their nails, but some complain of the opposite. This is likely due to the many vitamins and minerals being diverted to the developing fetus. If your nails do become weak, brittle, dry or dull, you are probably low in certain nutrients or not absorbing them properly. Nails need the B-complex vitamins and Vitamins C, A, E (alpha tocoph-erol), and D. They also need protein, calcium, zinc, iodine, and iron. If these nutrients are not sufficiently supplied, the body will rob the nails to provide for the growing baby.

Great Sex

In the second trimester blood flow to the pelvic area increases, breasts are larger and more sensitive, and hormones are high, resulting in increased libido, greater sensitivity to sex, and better, stronger orgasms. During this period, you'll probably feel like having sex a little more or even a whole lot more. Take advantage of the situation! Once the baby is born, there will be little time or energy for sex, at least for awhile.

Reduced Breast Cancer Risk

Pregnancy and breastfeeding have been associated with reduced risk of breast cancer later in life. There are a few pregnancy-related factors behind this protection:

+ Early age at the full first term pregnancy
+ Multiple births
+ Preeclampsia
+ Long-term breastfeeding

Genetic Changes in the Breast's Cells

The breast is composed of a few different types of cells: lobular cells 1, 2, 3, and 4; duct cells; and fat cells. The breast's lobular type 1 cells actually change their genetic structure and protect women from estrogen-positive cancer—particularly those women who were pregnant before the age of 20. According to Dr. Kathleen T. Ruddy, author of the blog BreastCancerByDrRuddy, "A full-term pregnancy produces permanent genetic and biologic changes in the breast. And if the first full-term pregnancy occurs prior to age twenty, these permanent changes produce a life-time reduction in the risk for estrogen-positive breast cancer, the most common form of the disease (80 percent.)"

Researchers are not certain exactly why the lobular type 1 cell transfor-mation occurs but they are aware of two hormones that help provide the protection. "Estriol appears to alter the genetic profile of normal breast cells, making them more stable and resistant to malignant transformation," says Dr. Ruddy. "The other hormone that may play a role in protecting lobular type 1 cells is HCG, human chorionic gonadatropin, also produced in very high quantities during pregnancy."

Lowered Estrogen Levels Over a Lifetime

Here's another upside to breastfeeding: Mothers who do it for an extended period of time—over one to two years, and especially with twins or triplets—reduces her risk of breast cancer. A woman's exposure to estrogen over a lifetime can put her at greater risk of developing breast cancer. And women who have had more menstrual periods—meaning they started menstruating earlier in life or went through menopause later in life—seem to be at a greater risk of developing breast cancer. Pregnancy and long-term breastfeeding significantly reduce the risk because they put a temporary halt on estrogen production. From the website of the American Cancer Society:

> *"Pregnancy causes many hormone changes in the body. For one thing, pregnancy stops the monthly menstrual cycles and shifts the hormone balance toward progesterone rather than estrogen. This is why women who become pregnant while they are young and have many pregnancies may have a slightly lower risk of breast cancer later on. Women who have had no children or who had their first pregnancy after age 30 have a slightly higher breast cancer risk later in life."*

In addition to protection against breast cancer, pregnancy and breastfeeding also lower the risk of endometrial cancer and ovarian cancer. It seems as though women were designed to have children. The body is more susceptible to breaking down when we don't live as nature intended.

That Stellar Sense of Smell

Some women consider it a drawback. Me, I thought my heightened sense of smell was the coolest thing ever! Most women complain about this during the first trimester, when certain smells become noxious. There is definitely a link between food and smell aversions, but while it's easy to avoid eating foods you don't like, it's a harder to avoid smells. To me, it's a glass half-full kind of thing: Maybe some smells get worse, but think of all the wonderful smells you never noticed or had the opportunity to enjoy before now? I lived in California during my first pregnancy and my house backed up against a creek trail. Between February and December there was always some flower in bloom. Walking down that trail each day was such a treat—one of my favorite things about pregnancy.

There are benefits to this seemingly random symptom. In fact, your heightened sense of smell is a protective mechanism designed to keep potentially poisonous foods or substances away from the growing fetus. There is a good reason why some perfumes, air fresheners like Febreeze, and scented candles can smell nauseating to pregnant women: They all contain toxic chemicals and synthetic hormones!

So think of your enhanced sense of smell as a useful tool. If something stinks, steer clear of it. This goes for foods, too. Some fruits, like peaches, often contain high amounts of pesticides. If you've developed an aversion to peaches, maybe your body is trying to protect the baby from chemicals. A pregnant woman's sense of smell is one of the first of many motherly instincts designed by nature to protect her child.

Rib Expansion

A pregnant woman's ribs must expand somewhat to accommodate the baby in the last trimester. This can mean aching ribs, especially if the baby is breech. If you suffer from this, get on all fours; you'll notice near total relief from rib pain. Four legged animals really do have the advantage when it comes to pregnancy.

Your body is making room for the baby but it is also expanding your rib cage to provide space for greater lung capacity. A pregnant woman is able to take in 30-40 percent more air through her lungs, which is important for delivering oxygen to the baby. But the expansion is not just for respiration: pregnant women *lose* some breathing capacity due to the compression and displacement of the diaphragm by the fetus. So in the end, inspiratory capacity only increases by 5-10 percent.

There are plenty of women who experience no significant discomfort as the body makes room for the baby. The hormones that loosen ligaments can render the gradual adjustments painless. Nevertheless, some of us do. To help ease discomfort, focus on maintaining good posture. Sitting down can be the most uncomfortable position; standing, walking, and resting on all fours might offer relief. Stretching the arms above the head and even practicing yoga or another stretching routine will help keep the body loose.

So, after all this talk about the problems of rib expansion why is it in this chapter about advantages? Because after the baby is born the ribs sometimes remain slightly expanded, giving mothers a slightly greater lung capacity. Bigger breaths not only alkalize the body (anesthesiologists are aware of this because during labor alkalosis is a threat), they help deliver oxygen to every cell. Deep breathing calms the mind and can even aid in the treatment of mental disorders.

And as a singer, greater lung capacity means sustaining notes for longer. The phenomenon is anecdotal but the belief is common among singers that ribs remain slightly expanded after pregnancy. And that allows them to produce larger and more sustained sounds. Before a breath is even taken a singer will sort of open her ribs to make room for the in and out movement of the lungs. If the ribs really do remain in a slightly outward position after childbirth, this gives a singer like myself a little advantage. I may look a little bonier, but my technique is much better!

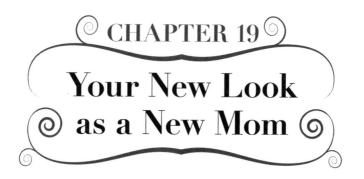

CHAPTER 19

Your New Look as a New Mom

We've established how pregnancy and childbirth have the power to change the way you look. It also has the power to change the way you think and act. A new mother undergoes psychological transformations more profound than any other she may ever experience. Forevermore, she will be different from her non-mother female friends, much like a world traveler is different from someone who has never left his own backyard.

All of the major events in our lives shape us. Being a college student, for example, guides our influences, our fears, our hopes. Taking a year to backpack alone through foreign countries opens a person up to challenges and new ways of thinking. But motherhood is bigger than travel, school, career, and marriage. Becoming a mother forces us to give up certain aspects of ourselves in exchange for others. The change is permanent and unconditional. Mothers adopt a new lifestyle that, for most of us, could never have happened without the responsibility and love that another life brings.

When the Changes of Motherhood Begin

The switch from womanhood to motherhood begins in pregnancy, is solidified at the birth of the baby, and grows throughout each stage of a child's development.

Pregnancy

Just the idea that we are making a person in our bellies is powerful enough to inspire a woman to change her diet, give up alcohol and cigarettes, change her personal care products, and start eating organic. These may be changes she's been struggling to implement for a long time, and now, somehow, it comes easily.

Later in pregnancy, the feeling of this little human life kicking inside conjures up the love that will soon grow so large. We take the discomforts in stride and put up with it all for someone we haven't even met yet.

Birth

Labor is hard work, whether you have adopted a Primal path or not. Remember, we're not well-designed birthing machines (more like sex machines with brains). The hours of discomfort, pain, and concentration during labor catapults a woman into a whole new life with many more demands. But it is seeing, hearing, smelling, and touching the baby for the first time that crystalizes all of the preparation that has been in progress for the last nine months.

The directed movements of the baby's head and eyes toward its mother's face establishes a bond more intimate than any she has known. Sooner after, the baby searches for her mother's nipple. For this newborn, there is only one person in the world who matters. The mother has been chosen and she must confidently assume the role as primary caretaker.

The Changes That Take Place

Having a child elicits both gradual and dramatic changes. There is no greater challenge a woman can face. As a result, she will become stronger, more responsible, a better problem solver and multitasker. The helplessness of the baby will make her more caring, and her worries over the health of her child will distract her from unessential preoccupations. The way she views her role within her family will change too.

Love Will Change Her

Regardless of how many good relationships a woman has been in and how much love she has felt for those people, she will find that the love for her baby is stronger than any love she's ever known. If she has never loved or been loved before, she will experience this, profoundly, for the first time.

Strength Will Change Her

The confidence and accomplishment that a woman experiences after laboring and giving birth changes her perception of herself. She now sees herself as someone who can withstand the impossible. She is stronger than she has ever been before.

Her Worries and Focus Will Change

A mother cannot let her baby starve, drown, fall, catch a cold, bang its head, suffocate, freeze, or overheat. She is motivated and moved by these possibilities. They keep her vigilant. She may become obsessive and possessive as a result of these worries. She may become overwhelmed. She may become overprotective. A woman who used to be shy or reserved may find herself suddenly bold or presumptuous.

Her Status Will Change

A mother's new responsibilities forced her to reorder her role in her family, in her home, with her friends. She is the boss of someone now, if she wasn't before. Her parents stop seeing her as a child. Her relationships with old friends may end, but new friendships will begin. As her attention is increasingly drawn to her baby, she will become less concerned with the way she looks; she might even dress differently. Her interests and activities will evolve, too.

Her Job Will Change

Mothers are protectors and enablers. It is their job to keep a child safe all day and night. It is also her job to assist the child in becoming the person he or she will be. She will do this job every day for the rest of her life.

How Motherhood Changes Us

Parenting changes us by challenging our weaknesses. For each of us this will mean something different. For me it was becoming less selfish and solitary. For others it's becoming healthier or more loving. We can't know what will change before it happens. That's one of the exciting things about motherhood. We will change but we won't know how until it happens.

I asked some of the mothers who visit my blog to tell me about their own changes. I got some remarkable answers.

* Diane's children made her selfless. "Being a mother is the epitome of evolution. I have evolved from a self-centered, career-driven, globe-trotter into a woman who derives joy from watching her children discover all the fascinating nuances of the world around them... The admiration and approval (hugs and kisses) of toddlers is so much more

gratifying than any glowing professional review I have received. I would sacrifice anything for my children."

* Sam educated herself and quickly made better lifestyle choices. She said that she started learning about health and nutrition right around the time she got pregnant. And after her daughter was born she "got on the fast track of being aware of what our family puts in our bodies and making a conscious effort to raise our family in a healthy way."

* Jamie found profound strength during labor. Her birth didn't go as planned and while she wanted a home birth, she ended up in the hospital. They weren't very friendly to her 'hippy" ways and were condescending at every turn. Before her stay in the maternity ward she "used to cower in the face of doctors, thinking they knew best. I would ignore my own body in favor of their words. After my birth, I grew a phenomenal inner fortitude. I will fight tooth and nail, to my death, for what I know is right for me and my child. And if you get in my way, I know I can kick you right down. To the floor, if I have to. I know this because I did."

* Jamie also said that she sold her piano to pay for her midwife. As a piano player myself, I have to say that's dedication! When I asked her if she ever got a new one, she said, "Not yet. Turns out having a child transformed my bank account more than my soul." We can all relate to that. She supports herself and her son in San Francisco through a modest business called Oh Crap Potty Training. She's got some pretty sound advice in her book of the same title. When you're ready to get your kid out of diapers, you might want to help her get that piano back.

* Michelle became more responsible as a result of her child's keen awareness. "It sounds cliché, but having a child made me really and truly want to be a better person... for my daughter." She said that seeing her child imitate her put her choices in the spotlight and made her realize that being a good example is so important. "I see how she internalizes everything she sees me do and copies it. If she were to see me eating Oreos and Doritos all day long, that is what she would want to do too."

* And if you wonder how a child can change a woman so dramatically, even when she's spent her life caught up in herself, listen to Sarah. "I worried too about being selfish and giving up my lifestyle, but have found that it's that exact selfishness that lets you be a great caretaker

for your child, because it's just an extension of yourself, another part of YOU (not some person that you don't know). You'll selfishly turn down your friends and your hobbies for your child because it's you."

Why Does Motherhood Change Us?

Why is motherhood different from being a sister, or daughter, or wife, or friend? Why do we rise to the challenge? Why don't we seem to have a choice?

Because of instinct. Because it's what makes us human. Because it's Primal.

Nothing is more instinctual than reproduction. Nothing is more distinctly human than to expend every possible effort for the success of our offspring. And nothing is more Primal than to recognize and follow those instincts.

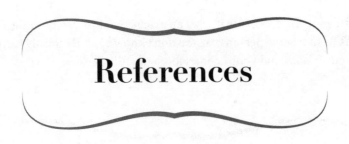

References

CHAPTER 1
What it Means To Be Primal

1. **The Paleo Diet**, *Loren Cordain (defining paleo)*

2. **The Primal Blueprint**, *Mark Sisson (defining primal)*

3. **Nutrition and health in agriculturalists and hunter-gatherers: a case study of two prehistoric populations**, *Eds Jerome NW et al., Nutritional Anthropology, 1980 Redgrave Publishing Company, Pleasantville, NY pg 117-145 (comparing hunter gatherers and agriculturists)*

4. **Hunter-gatherer diets—a different perspective**, *Katharine Milton, American* Journal of Clinical Nutrition, Vol. 71, No. 3, 665-667, March 2000 http://www.ajcn.org/content/71/3/665.full#R11 (regardless of source of dietary energy, hunter-gatherers thrived, Katharine Milton quoted)

5. **Colas but not other carbonated beverages, are associated with low bone mineral density in older women: The Framingham Osteoporosis Study**, Katharine L Tucker et all, American Journal of Clinical Nutrition, Vol. 84, No. 4, 936-942, October 2006 (soda leaches calcium from the bones)

6. ***Effects of Stress***, *American Institute of Stress*, http://www.stress.org/topic-effects.htm (symptoms of stress)

7. **The Age-Free Zone**, Dr. Barry Sears (*prostaglandin production and immune health*)

CHAPTER 3
Fertility, Conception, and Child Spacing

8. **Pottenger's Cats**, Francis M Pottenger (effects of nutrition on subsequent generations)

9. **Fast Stats—Infertility**, CDC website http://www.cdc.gov/nchs/fastats/fertile.htm (infertility statistics)

10. **Vitamin D—roles in women's reproductive health?**, Grundmann M, et all, Reprod Biol Endocrinol. 2011, http://www.rbej.com/content/9/1/146 (Vitamin D)

11. **Fertility Diet**, Chevarro, Willett, and Skerrett, 134 (iron is needed by the egg to make protein and DNA)

12. **On the Trail of the Elusive X-Factor**, Chris Masterjojn, http://www.westonaprice.org/fat-soluble-activators/x-factor-is-vitamin-k2 (K2 and infant growth)

13. **Vitamin C Increases Fertility in Women with Luteal Phase Defect**, Healthnotes, http://www.bastyrcenter.org/content/view/620/ (improves fertility in women with luteal phase defect)

14. **Vitamin C Prevents Premature Birth,** Healthnotes, http://www.bastyrcenter.org/content/view/632/#top (prevents preterm birth)

15. **The Little Known (but crucial) Difference Between Folate and Folic Acid,** Chris Kresser, http://chriskresser.com/folate-vs-folic-acid (folic acid)

16. **Real Food for Mother and Baby**, Nina Plank (fertility nutrients)

17. **Bee Propolis May Improve Fertility in Women with Endometriosis,** Healthnotes, http://www.bastyrcenter.org/content/view/623/#top (bee propolis)

18. **The placenta really does act like a parasite, Reading research suggests**, University of Reading press release, 2007, http://www.reading.ac.uk/news-and-events/releases/PR9938.aspx (how the placenta works)

19. **Deep Nutrition: Why Your Genes Need Traditional Food**, Catherine Shanahan (facial structure, second sibling syndrome)

20. **Natural Causes: Death, Lies, and Politics in America's Vitamin and Herbal Supplement Industry**, Dan Hurly, Broadway 2006 (supplements)

21. **Beyond Deficiency: New Views on the Function and Health Effects of Vitamins**, Annals of the New York Academy of Sciences, Vol 669, 1992, Pp8-10 (supplements)

CHAPTER 4
Eating For the Primal Pregnancy

22. **Woolly Mammoth Carcass May Have Been Cut Into By Humans**, BBC Nature reporter Ben Avis, http://www.bbc.co.uk/nature/17525070 (Most recent evidence to support the theory that early humans were scavengers and not hunters)

23. **Absorption of heme iron**, Semin Hematol. 1998 Jan;35(1):27-34, Uzel C, Comrad ME, http://www.ncbi.nlm.nih.gov/pubmed/9460807, (heme iron absorbed better than plant iron)

24. **Bioavailability of iron,** Hurrell RF, American Journal of Clinical Nutrition, 1997;51(S);1:S4-S8, http://www.ajcn.org/content/91/5/1461S.full

25. **Guts and Grease: the diet of Native American Indians**, Sally Fallon and Mary G. Enig PhD, http://www.westonaprice.org/traditional-diets/guts-and-grease (diet of Native Americans)

26. **Chemicals in Meats Cooked at High Temperatures and Cancer Risk,** National Cancer Institute Fact Sheet, http://www.cancer.gov/cancertopics/factsheet/Risk/cooked-meats (carcinogens in overcooked meat)

27. http://www.heart.org/HEARTORG/GettingHealthy/FatsAndOils/MeettheFats/Meet-the-Fats_UCM_304495_Article.jsp (what the AMA has to say about fats)

28. **The Skinny on Fats,** Mary G. Enig PhD and Sally Fallon, http://www.westonaprice.org/know-your-fats/skinny-on-fats (cholesterol, benefits of saturated fat, source of fat-soluble vitamins)

29. **The Benefits of High Cholesterol**, Uffe Ravinskov, http://www.we-stonaprice.org/cardiovascular-disease/benefits-of-high-cholesterol (cholesterol's important role in the body)

30. **The Cholesterol Conundrum**, by the Psychology Today staff, Psychology Today, May 1, 1995, http://www.psychologytoday.com/articles/199505/the-cholesterol-conundrum (cholesterol makes you happier)

31. **The Effects of Fat and Cholesterol on Social Behavior in Monkeys** JAY R. KAPLAN, PHD, STEPHEN B. MANUCK, PHD, AND CAROL SHIVELY, PHD, Psychosomatic Medicine 53:634-642 (1991)

32. **What Causes heart Disease**, Sally Fallon and Mary Enig PhD http://www.westonaprice.org/cardiovascular-disease/what-causes-heart-disease (the real cause of heart disease)

33. **Leading Causes of Death 1900-1998**, Centers for Disease Control and Prevention http://www.cdc.gov/nchs/data/dvs/lead1900_98.pdf (heart disease statistics)

34. **The Trouble With Fructose: A Darwinian Perspective**, talk given by Dr. Robert Lustig, http://vimeo.com/29402977 (limit fruit)

35. **Dietary fiber and mineral bioavailability,** Harland BF, Nutrition Research Reviews 1989; 2:133-47, http://journals.cambridge.org/download.php?file=%2FNRR%2FNRR2_01%2FS0954422489000120a.pdf&code=f8486fae8dd725985695a37a3d8fa71f

36. **Dietary Fiber Intake Increases the Risk of Zinc Deficiency in Healthy and Diabetic Women**, Foster M et all, Biological Trace Element Research, 2012 April 21, http://www.ncbi.nlm.nih.gov/pubmed/22528778 (phyitic acid and fiber inhibits mineral absorption)

37. **Deep Nutrition: Why Your Genes Need Traditional Food**, Catherine Shanahan (fermentation)

38. **Living With Phytic Acid**, Ramiel Nagel, http://www.westonaprice.org/food-features/living-with-phytic-acid (phytic acid in nuts and seeds)

39. **Inhibitory Effects of Nuts on Iron Absorption**, Bruce J Macfarlan et. all, American Journal of Clinical Nutrition, Vol 47, 270-274, 1988 (nuts and phytic acid)

40. **Common Neonatal Infections,** KidsHealth.org, http://kidshealth. org/parent/infections/common/neonatal_infections.html# (infections contracted during birth)

41. **Oats as Feed for Beef Cattle, LaDon Johnson and Stephan Boyles, North Dakota State University,** http://www.ag.ndsu.edu/pubs/an-sci/beef/as1020w.htm (cattle feed)

42. **The Untold Story of Milk**, Ron Schmid (milk facts)

43. **Protein and Calcium: antagonists or synergists**, Robert P. Heaney, American Journal of Clinical Nutrition, Vol. 75, No. 4, 609-610, April 2002 http://www.ajcn.org/content/75/4/609.full (high protein and calcium absorption)

44. **Micronutrient Information Center**, Calcium, Linus Pauling Institute, http://lpi.oregonstate.edu/infocenter/minerals/calcium/index. html

45. **National Academies Press, Seafood Safety Executive Summary** http://www.nap.edu/openbook.php?record_id=1612&page=1 (quote, "Most seafood-associated illness…" page 1, and "cross-contamination of cooked by raw product" page 8, plus info on parasites and types of fish)

46. Gut Bacteria Regulate Happiness, John F Cryan, news@ucc (brand new unpublished research on the link between gut microbes and serotonin)

47. http://www.homebrew.net/ferment/#yeast (alcohol fermentation)

48. Fetal Alcohol Syndrome, National Library of Medicine, A.D.A.M. Medical Encyclopedia http://www.ncbi.nlm.nih.gov/pubmed-health/PMH0001909/ (fetal alcohol syndrome symptoms)

49. **Farm management choice can benefit fungi key to healthy ecosystems**, Centre for Hydrology and Ecology, http://www.ceh.ac.uk/ news/news_archive/2010_news_item_31.html (lack of chemicals in soil enables microbial diversity)

50. **Nutritional quality of organic versus conventional fruits, vegetables, and grains**, Worthington V, J Altern Complement Med. 2001 Apr;7(2):161-73,

51. **EWG's Shoppers Guide to Pesticides in Produce**, Environmental Working Group Executive summary, http://www.ewg.org/food-news/summary/ (the dirty dozen)

CHAPTER 5
The Importance Of Diet On Baby's Gene Expression

52. **Nutrition and Physical Degeneration**, Weston A. Price, A Project Gutenberg of Australia eBook, eBook No.: 0200251h.html, Chapter 21, http://gutenberg.net.au/ebooks02/0200251h.html#ch21 (Weston A. Price quotes)

53. **Genes and Chromosomes: The Genome**, Center for Genetics Education, http://www.genetics.edu.au/Information/Genetics-Fact-Sheets/Genes-and-Chromosomes-FS1 (genetics basics)

54. http://learn.genetics.utah.edu/ (basic genetics)

55. **Environmental factors can alter the way our genes are expressed, making even identical twins different**, NOVA, aired 7/24/07 on PBS, http://www.pbs.org/wgbh/nova/body/epigenetics.html (Randy Jirtle quoted)

56. **Epigenetics Means What We Eat, How We Live and Love, Alters How Our Genes Behave**, By Duke Medicine News and Communications, http://www.dukehealth.org/health_library/news/9322 (David Barker quoted)

57. **Epigenetic Gene Promoter Methylation at Birth is Associated With Child's Later Adiposity**, Keith M Godfrey et all, http://diabetes.diabetesjournals.org/content/early/2011/04/04/db10-0979.abstract (early gene methylation and obesity)

58. **Dietary prenatal choline supplementation alters postnatal hippocampal structure and function**, Li Q, et all, Journal of Neurophysiology, 2004 http://www.ncbi.nlm.nih.gov/pubmed/14645379 (methylation, choline in rats)

59. **A Thing or Two About Twins**, Peter Miller, National Geographic, January 2012, http://ngm.nationalgeographic.com/2012/01/twins/miller-text (epigenetic differences between identical twins)

60. **Nutrition and the Epigenome**, University of Utah, http://learn.genetics.utah.edu/content/epigenetics/nutrition/ (specific methyl-donating nutrients)

CHAPTER 6
Exercise During and After Pregnancy

61. **Exercising Through Your Pregnancy**, James F. Clapp III MD, Addicus Books; 1 edition, January 2002 (main resource)

62. **The Truth About Prenatal Exercise**, http://www.fitpregnancy. com/workouts/prenatal-workouts/truth-about-prenatal-exercise (prenatal exercise myths)

63. **Climbing, Exercising and Pregnancy: A Reality Check**, http:// www.bodyresults.com/e2pregnancyexercise.asp (extreme sports and pregnancy)

64. **Exercise After Pregnancy: How to Look and Feel Your Best**, Helene Byrne Be-fit Mom, 2nd edition, June 2007 (alignment)

CHAPTER 7
Stretch Marks

65. **Micronutrients and Skin Health**, Linus Pauling Institute http:// lpi.oregonstate.edu/infocenter/skin.html (layers of the skin, wound healing, skin nutrition, quote)

66. **Striae gravidarum in primiparae**, Atwal, G.S.S., Manku, L.K., Griffiths, C.E.M. and Polson, D.W. British Journal of Dermatology, 155: 965-969. doi: 10.1111/j.1365-2133.2006.07427.x, (study on incidence in younger women)

67. **Risk factors associated with striae gravidarum**, Chang AL, Agredano YZ, Kimball AB., J Am Acad Dermatol. 2004 Dec;51(6):881-5(ethnicity)

68. **Proteoglycans and Glycosaminoglycans**, Chapter 11 contributed by J.D. Esko Essentials of Glycobiology, 2nd eduition, Chapter 11, http://www.ncbi.nlm.nih.gov/books/NBK20693/ (properties of glycosaminoglycans)

69. **Prevention of Sriae gravidarum with cocoa butter cream**, Keisha Buchanan et all, International Journal of Gynecology Obstetrics, September 2009 (cocoa butter findings)

70. **Prophylaxis of Striae gravidarum with a topical formulation. A double blind trial**, Mallol J et all, International Journal of Cosmetic Science, 1991 Feb;13(1):51-7

71. **Vital Chi Skin Brushing System,** Bruce Berkowsky, Joseph Ben Hil-Meyer Research Press, September 2011

72. **Vitamin A antagonizes decreased cell growth and elevated collagen-degrading matrix metalloproteinases and stimulates collagen accumulation in naturally aged human skin,** Varani J et all, Journal of Investigative Dermatology. 2000 Mar;114(3):480-6. (Vitamin A applications stimulate collagen formation)

73. **Vitamin C and Skin Health,** Linus Pauling Institute, http://lpi. oregonstate.edu/infocenter/skin/vitaminC/index.html (benefits of topical Vitamin C)

CHAPTER 8
Cellulite

74. **The Cellulite Solution**, Howard Murad, M.D., St. Martins Press, 2005 (water principle of cellulite)

75. **Cellulite Anatomy**, Cellulite Skincare and Cellulite Expert Academy http://www.celluliteexpert.com/english/cellulite.html (anatomy)

76. **Cellulite Profile**, Cellulite Skincare and Cellulite Expert Academy http://www.celluliteexpert.com/english/profile.html (measuring cellulite)

77. **Molecular Biology of the Cell, Chapter: The Extracellular Matrix of the Cell,** Alberts B, Johnson A, Lewis J, et al, 4th edition, New York: Garland Science; 2002. (extracellular matrix)

78. **Silent Waves: Theory and Practice of Lymph Drainage Therapy,** Bruno Chikly, MD, DO (lymph)

79. **The Immune System Cure,** Lorna R Vanderhaeghe and Patrick J.D. Bouic, PhD, Kensington books, 1999 (lymphatic system)

80. Fat Flush Plan, Ann Louise Gittleman, McGraw Hill, 2002 (toxic liver)

81. **Blog talk radio at Underground Wellness**, with Cate Shanahan, 01/08/2011, http://www.blogtalkradio.com/undergroundwell-ness/2011/01/08/more-deep-nutrition-with-dr-cate-shanahan (overcooked meats and cellulite)

82. **THE ROLE OF FLUORIDE IONS IN GLYCOSAMINOGLYCANS SULPHATION IN CULTURED FIBROBLASTS**, Katarzyna Pawlowska-Goral et all, Fluoride Vol. 31 No. 4 193-202 1998. Research Report 193 http://www.fluorideresearch.org/314/files/FJ1998_v31_n4_p193-202.pdf (fluoride and connective tissue)

83. **The Best Cellulite Treatment—A Holistic Approach**, Marcelle Pick, OB/GYN NP, article at http://www.womentowomen.com/detoxification/cellulite.aspx (page 2 cellulite and toxins)

84. **Enzyme Nutrition**, Dr. Edward Howell, Avery Publishing Group, January 1995

85. **The Cellulite Cure**, Dr. Lionel Bissoon (lymph theory of cellulite)

86. **Effects and Side-Effects of 2% Progesterone Cream on the Skin of Peri- and Postmenopausal Women: Results from a Double-Blind, Vehicle-Controlled, Randomized Study**, Gregor Holzer, M.D., et al., British Journal of Dermatology August 2005

CHAPTER 9
Varicose Veins and Hemorrhoids

87. **The Cellulite Solution**, Howard Murad, M.D., St. Martins Press, 2005

88. **The Fiber Menace**, Konstantin Monastyrsky (constipation and hemorrhoids)

89. **Vein**, from Encyclopedia Britannica, http://www.britannica.com/EBchecked/topic/624704/vein

90. **Blood Vessel**, Encyclopedia Britannica, http://www.britannica.com/EBchecked/topic/69887/blood-vessel

91. **Varicose Vein**, Encyclopedia Britannica, http://www.britannica.com/EBchecked/topic/623435/varicose-vein

92. **Varicose Veins,** Stanford Hospital and Clinics http://stanfordhospital.org/clinicsmedServices/COE/surgicalServices/vascularSurgery/patientEducation/varicose.html

CHAPTER 10
Split Abdominal Muscles—Diastasis Recti

93. **Incidence of Diastasis Recti Abdominis During the Childbearing Year,** Jill Schiff Boissonnault and Mary Jo Blaschak, Physical Therapy: Journal of the American Physical Therapy Association, 1988; 68:1082-1086. (research)

94. **Moms Into Fitness blog,** Lidsay Brin, Author of the Moms Into Fitness fitness DVDs, http://www.momsintofitness.com/faq-flat-stomachs-and-diastasis-recti(exercises, techniques, test)

95. **Abdominal muscle,** Encyclopedia Britannica http://www.britannica.com/EBchecked/topic/867/abdominal-muscle#ref82763 (anatomy)

96. **The One-Leg Standing Test and the Active Straight Leg Raise Test: A Clinical Interpretation of Two Tests of Load Transfer through the Pelvic Girdle,** Diane G. Lee, Linda-Joy Lee, Orthopaedic Division Review - 2005 http://www.kalindra.com/LoadTransfertests.pdf (test for diastasis recti)

97. **Diastasis rectus abdominis & postpartum health,** Diane Lee and Associates http://dianelee.ca/education/article_diastasis.php (surgical repair)

98. **Lose Your Mummy Tummy,** Julie Tupler and Jodie Gould, Da Capo Press, 2004 (Tupler Technique for minimizing diastasis)

99. **Dialogue with Ann Wendel of Prana Physical Therapy** (exercises, quotes, pictures)

CHAPTER 11
Sagging Breasts and Vaginal Dryness

100. **Slide show: Female Breast Anatomy,** The Mayo Clinic, http://www.mayoclinic.com/health/breast-cancer-early-stage/BC00001 (anatomy of the breast)

101. **Pectoralis Muscles,** Encyclopedia Britannica, http://www.britannica.com/EBchecked/topic/448397/pectoralis-muscle

102. **Exercises That Lift Saggy Breasts,** Rose Erikson on Livestrong.com, http://www.livestrong.com/article/389454-exercises-that-lift-saggy-breasts/

103. **Vagina,** Encyclopedia Britannica, http://www.britannica.com/EBchecked/topic/621487/vagina (anatomy)

104. **Menopause Matters: Your Guide to a Long and Healthy Life,** Julia Schlam Edelmen, Johns Hopkins University Press, 2009 (vaginal dryness and quote)

CHAPTER 12
Foods and Supplements To Support Connective Tissue

105. **Dietary Supplement Fact Sheet: Iron,** Office of Dietary Supplements, National Institutes of Health, http://ods.od.nih.gov/factsheets/iron

106. **Perfect Hormone Balance For Pregnancy,** Dr. Robert Greene, Three Rivers Press, 2007

107. **Molecular Biology of the Cell, Chapter: The Extracellular Matrix of the Cell,** Alberts B, Johnson A, Lewis J, et al, 4th edition, New York: Garland Science; 2002.

108. **Effect of catechin on connective tissue,** Bloomenkrantz N, Asboe-Hansen G. Scand J Rheumatol, 1978;7:55-60

CHAPTER 13
Protruding, Sagging Belly

109. **Prenatal and Postpartum Exercise Design**, by Catherine Cram, M.S., and Gwen Hyatt, M.S., Copyright 2003,

110. Exercise After Pregnancy, How to Look and Feel Your Best, Helene Byrne, Celestial Arts, 2001

CHAPTER 14
Weight Gain

111. **Why does fat deposit on the hips and buttocks of women and around the stomachs of men?**, Patrick J Bird, Scientific American, May 15, 2006 http://www.scientificamerican.com/article.cfm?id=why-does-fat-deposit-on-t (placement of fat and hormones)

112. **Weight Gain in Pregnancy—Past, Present, and Future**, Naomi E. Stotland, MD, Dept. of Obstetrics, Gynecology, and Reproductive Sciences, UCSF (history of weight gain)

113. **How Much Weight Gain is Healthy During Pregnancy?**, Yvonne Thornton, MD, Huffington Post, 2/24/11, http://www.huffingtonpost.com/yvonne-thornton-md/pregnancy-weight-gain-b_824894.html (old weight gain recommendations)

114. **Pregnancy Weight Gain,** Web MD Medical Reference, Reviewed by Mikio A. Nihira, MD on March 07, 2010, http://www.webmd.com/baby/guide/healthy-weight-gain (new weight gain recommendations)

115. **The million-year wait for macroevolutionary bursts**, Josef C. Uyeda et al, PNAS 2011 108 (38) 15908-15913; published ahead of print August 23, 2011, doi:10.1073/pnas.1014503108 (evolutionary changes in physiology)

116. **Pregnancy weight gain and breast cancer risk**, Kinnunen TI, et al, BMC Women's Health. 2004 Oct 21;4(1):7 (women who gain excess weight during pregnancy at higher risk of developing breast cancer)

117. **Mother's Pregnancy Weight Linked to Child's Obesity,** Katherine Harmon, August 5, 2010, http://www.scientificamerican.com/article.cfm?id=mothers-pregnancy-weight (David Ludwig obesity study and Dr. Ludwig quote)

118. **Estrogen Imprinting: When Your Epigenetic Memories Come Back to Haunt You,** Endocrinology 149(12):5919-5921, Printed in U.S.A. Copyright 2008 by The endocrine Society, doi: 10.1210/en.2008-1266 (hormonal imprinting)

119. **The Fat Resistance Diet**, Leo Galland, MD, Broadway Books, copyright 2005 (inflammation)

120. **Vitamin D and Weight Loss**, Website: vitamin D deficiency symptoms guide, http://www.vitaminddeficiencysymptomsguide.com/vitamin-d-and-weight-loss/ (Vitamin D and weight loss)

121. **The Nutritional Deficiency That Will Prevent Weight Loss—Even With Diet and Exercise**, website: unconventional health http://www.unconventionalhealth.com/Nutritional-Deficiency-Prevents-Weight-Loss.html (iodine, thyroid, and weight loss)

122. **Bugs Inside: What Happens When the Microbes That Keep Us Healthy Disappear?**, Katherine Harmon, Scientific American, December 16, 2009, http://www.scientificamerican.com/article.cfm?id=human-microbiome-change (change in human microbiome)

123. **A Healthy Gut is the Hidden Key to Weight Loss**, Chris Kresser, October 29, 2010, http://thehealthyskeptic.org/a-healthy-gut-is-the-hidden-key-to-weight-loss (gut health)

124. **Human gut microbes associated with obesity**, Ruth E Lee, et. al, Microbial Biology, Nature Publishing Group, 2006, http://gordon-lab.wustl.edu/PublicationPDFs/370_LeyNature06.pdf (quote)

125. **Short Sleep Duration Is Associated with Reduced Leptin, Elevated Ghrelin, and Increased Body Mass Index**, Shahrad Taheri et al, http://www.plosmedicine.org/article/info%3Adoi%2F10.1371%2Fjournal.pmed.0010062 (sleep and weight loss)

CHAPTER 15
Hair Loss, Hair Growth, and Your Skin

126. **Perfect Hormone Balance For Pregnancy**, Dr. Robert Greene, Three Rivers Press, 2007

127. **Wounds**, University of Maryland Medical Center Online Medical Reference, http://www.umm.edu/altmed/articles/wounds-000175.htm

128. **Vitamin C requirements in postoperative patients**, Alster TS, West TB., Dermatol Surg. 1998 Mar;24(3):331-4 (reduction in circulating white blood cell ascorbic acid levels in postoperative patients)

129. **Gentle Healing for Baby and Child**, Andrea Candee, Pocket Books, 2000

CHAPTER 16
Depression

130. **Perinatal depression: prevalence, risks, and the nutrition link--a review of the literature.**, Leung BM, Kaplan BJ., J Am Diet Assoc. 2009 Sep;109(9):1566-75. (prevalence of ante and postnatal depression)

131. **Postpartum Depression Demystified: An Essential Guide for Understanding and Overcoming the Most Common Complication after Childbirth**, Joyce A. Venis RNC, Da Capo Press March 2007 (symptoms, risk factors)

132. **Depression in Childbearing Women: When Depression Complicates Pregnancy,** Sheila M. Marcus, MD and Julie E. Heringhausen, BSN, Prim Care. 2009 March; 36(1): 151-ix.doi: 10.1016/j.pop.2008.10.011 (effects of depression on fetus and infant)

133. **Depressive symptoms during pregnancy: Impact on neuroendocrine and neonatal outcomes**, Sheila Marcus, Infant Behavior

and Development, Volume 34, Issue 1, February 2011, Pages 26-34, (stress hormones in infants of depressed mothers)

134. **Postpartum depression linked with preteen violence**, Dale Hay, PhD et al, Developmental Psychology, Vol. 39, No. 6 (postpartum depression and preteen violence)

135. **Effective treatment for postpartum depression is not sufficient to improve the developing mother-child relationship,** Forman DR, Dev Psychopathol. 2007 Spring;19(2):585-602. (risks of postpartum depression for infants)

136. **Postpartum Depression For Dummies**, Shoshana S. Bennett, For Dummies; 1 edition January 2007 (history, statistics, treatments)

137. **The Functions of Postpartum Depression,** Edward H. Hagen, Evolution and Human Behavior 20: 325-359, 1999, Elsevier Science Inc. (parental investment theory, evolutionary psychology) http://www.anth.ucsb.edu/projects/human/ppd.pdf

138. **A Natural Guide to Pregnancy and Postpartum Health: The first book by doctors that really addresses pregnancy recovery**, Dr. Dean Raffelock. Avery, 2003 (SSRIs, serotonin)

139. **High antenatal maternal anxiety is related to ADHD symptoms, externalizing problems, and anxiety in 8- and 9-year-olds**, Van den Bergh BR, Marcoen A., Child Dev. 2004 Jul-Aug;75(4):1085-97. (anxiety during pregnancy leads to ADHD in children)

140. **Progesterone Supplementation and the Prevention of Preterm Birth**, Errol R Norwitz, MD, PhD et al, Rev Obstet Gynecol. 2011 Summer; 4(2): 60-72. (how progesterone prevents preterm birth)

141. **Elevated brain monoamine oxidase A binding in the early postpartum period**, Julia Sacher, et al. Arch Gen Psychiatry. 2010 May;67(5):468-74. (drop in estrogen causes increase in MAOA)

142. **The Mood Cure**, Julia Ross, Penguin, December 2003 (nutrient deficiencies and neurotransmitters)

143. **Perinatal depression: prevalence, risks, and the nutrition link-a review of the literature**, Leung BM, Kaplan BJ., J Am Diet Assoc. 2009 Sep;109(9):1566-75. (Canadian researchers quoted)

144. **Bottle feeding simulates child loss: Postpartum depression and evolutionary medicine,** Gordon G. Gallup Jr et all, Department of Psychology, University at Albany, (bottle feeding)

145. **Magnesium and the Brain: The Original Chill Pill**, Emily Deans, M.D., Published on June 12, 2011 in Evolutionary Psychiatry (magnesium deficiency and depression)

146. **IBS, Fructose, Depression, Zinc, and Women**, Emily Deans on her blog Evolutionary Psychiatry, http://evolutionarypsychiatry. blogspot.com/2010/08/ibs-fructose-depression-zinc-and-women. html (zinc and depression)

147. **Yoga as a Complementary Treatment of Depression: Effects of Traits and Moods on Treatment Outcome,** David Shapiro et al., Published online 2007 February 28. doi: 10.1093/ecam/nel114

148. **Risk Indices Associated with the Insulin Resistance Syndrome, Cardiovascular Disease, and Possible Protection with Yoga: A Systematic Review**, Kim E. Innes et al. JABFM, 10.3122/ jabfm.18.6.491J Am Board Fam Med November-December 2005 vol. 18 no. 6 491-519

149. **Fructose Malabsorption is Associated with Decreased Plasma Tryptophan**, Scandinavian Journal of Gastroenterology, 2001, Vol. 36, No. 4 , Pages 367-371 (doi:10.1080/00365520117856), M. Ledochowski et al. (fructose malabsorption and tryptophan) http://informahealthcare.com/doi/abs/10.1080/00365520117856

150. **Malabsorption of carbohydrates and depression in children and adolescents**, Varea V, de Carpi JM et al, J Pediatr Gastroenterol Nutr. 2005 May;40(5):561-5 (lactose and fructose malabsorption and depression) http://www.ncbi.nlm.nih.gov/pubmed/15861016

151. **Serotonin Syndrom**, Pubmed Health, http://www.ncbi.nlm.nih. gov/pubmedhealth/PMH0004531/

152. **Selective Serotonin Reuptake Inhibitor Toxicity**, Tracy A Cushing, MD, MPH, FACEP, FAWM, Medscape Reference, http://www. britannica.com/EBchecked/topic/533189/selective-serotonin-reuptake-inhibitor (SSRI info)

153. **Antidepressant use during pregnancy and childhood autism spectrum disorders**, Croen LA, Grether JK, et al, Arch Gen Psychiatry. 2011 Nov;68(11):1104-12. doi: 10.1001/archgenpsychiatry.2011.73. Epub 2011 Jul 4. (autism and antidepressants study)

154. **How SSRIs Taken During Pregnancy and Lactation Can Affect Newborns**, CPMC Sutter Health, The Pediatric Page http://www.

cpmc.org/advanced/pediatrics/physicians/pedpage-307neo.html
(effects of SSRIs on the fetus)

CHAPTER 17
Strategies and Supplements for Hormone Balance

155. **Chronic Cholesterol Depletion Using Statin Impairs the Function and Dynamics of Human Serotonin 1A Receptors**, Sandeep Shrivastava, Thomas J. Pucadyil‡, Yamuna Devi Paila, Sourav Ganguly and Amitabha Chattopadhyay, Biochemistry, 2010, 49 (26), pp 5426-5435DOI: 10.1021/bi100276bPublication Date (Web): June 3, 2010 (cholesterol lowering drugs cause depression)

156. **Plasma cholesterol and depressive symptoms in older men**, R.E. Morgan, BS,L.A. Palinkas, PhD,E.L. Barrett-Connor, MD, D.L. Wingard, PhD Volume 341, Issue 8837, 9 January 1993, Pages 75-79Originally published as Volume 1, Issue 8837 (low plasma cholesterol is associated with depression in men)

157. **Depressive Symptoms, Social Support, and Lipid Profile in Healthy Middle-AgedWomen,** MYRIAM HORSTEN, M S C, SARAH P. WAMALA, M S C, AD VINGERHOETS, P H D, ANDKRISTINA ORTH-GOMER, MD, Psychosomatic Medicine September 1, 1997 vol. 59 no. 5 521-528 (low plasma cholesterol is associated with depression in women)

158. **Low cholesterol and violent crime**, Beatrice A Golomba, Håkan Stattind, Sarnoff Mednicka, Journal of Psychiatric ResearchVolume 34, Issues 4-5, July 2000, Pages 301-309 (low cholesterol is common in criminals)

159. **A Double-Blind, Placebo-Controlled Study of the Omega-3 Fatty Acid Docosahexaenoic Acid in the Treatment of Major Depression,** Lauren B. Marangell et al., Am J Psychiatry 2003;160:996-998. 10.1176/appi.ajp.160.5.996 (DHA and depression)

160. **Effect of maternal docosahexaenoic acid supplementation on postpartum depression and information processing**, Antolin M. Llorente, PhD et al., American Journal of Obstetrics & Gynecology-Volume 188, Issue 5 , Pages 1348-1353, May 2003 (DHA and postpartum depression)

161. **Effect of supplementation with selenium on postpartum depression: a randomized double-blind placebo-controlled trial,** Mokhber N, Namjoo M, et al., J Matern Fetal Neonatal Med. 2011 Jan;24(1):104-8. Epub 2010 Jun 8.

162. **Selenium,** from World's Healthiest Foods, http://www.whfoods.com/genpage.php?dbid=95&tname=nutrient#deficiencysymptoms (foods containing selenium)

163. **Vitamin D association with estradiol and progesterone in young women,** Knight JA et al., Cancer Causes Control. 2010 Mar;21(3):479-83. (Vitamin D reduces breast cancer risk)

164. **Vitamin D supplementation, 25-hydroxyvitamin D concentrations, and safety,** Reinhold Vieth, American Society for Clinical Nutrition (Vitamin D requirements and quote)

165. **Environmental factors that influence the cutaneousproduction of vitamin D13, Michael F Holick,** Am J C/in Nutr 1995;61(suppl):638S-45S. Printed in USA.© 1995 American Society for Clinical Nutrition (getting Vitamin D from the sun)

166. **Can a Tanning Bed Be Healthy?** Dr. Mercola, http://articles.mercola.com/sites/articles/archive/2006/11/11/can-a-tanning-bed-be-healthy.aspx (types of tanning beds and quote)

167. **Role of Vitamin D in Insulin Secretion and Insulin Sensitivity for Glucose Homeostasis,** Jessica A. Alvarez and Ambika Ashraf, Published online 2009 August 19. doi: 10.1155/2010/351385

168. **Acupuncture Increases Nocturnal Melatonin Secretion and Reduces Insomnia and Anxiety: A Preliminary Report,** D. Warren Spence, M.A., The Journal of Neuropsychiatry and Clinical Neurosciences 2004;16:19-28. 10.1176/appi.neuropsych.16.1.19 (acupuncture's efficacy and melatonin secretion)

CHAPTER 18
Desirable Physical Effects of Pregnancy

169. **Bipedalism,** Encyclopedia Britannica, http://www.britannica.com/EBchecked/topic/66275/bipedalism (examples of other bipedal animals)

170. **Prehistory of Sex,** Timothy Taylor, (quote page 39)

171. **Pregnancy and the risk of breast cancer**, Kara Britt, Alan Ashworth, and Matthew Smalley, Endocr Relat Cancer December 1, 2007 14 907-933 (review of protection from breast cancer in young women)

172. **How And Why Early Pregnancy Lowers Breast Cancer Risk**, From Dr. Kathleen T. Ruddy's Breast Cancer Blog, http://breastcancerbydrruddy.com/?p=2674 (quote and architecture of the breast)

173. **Parity, age at first and last birth, and risk of breast cancer: a population-based study in Sweden,** Lambe M et al., Breast Cancer Res Treat. 1996;38(3):305-11. (breast cancer risk and number of births)

174. **Pregnancy and Breast Cancer**, American Cancer Society, http://www.cancer.org/Cancer/BreastCancer/MoreInformation/pregnancy-and-breast-cancer (quote on levels of estrogen to progesterone)

175. **Breast cancer and breastfeeding: collaborative reanalysis of individual data from 47 epidemiological studies in 30 countries, including 50302 women with breast cancer and 96973 women without the disease,** Collaborative Group on Hormonal Factors in Breast Cancer, Lancet. 2002 Jul 20;360(9328):187-95. (breast feeding's effect on breast cancer)

176. **Physiological Changes Associated with Pregnancy, Respiratory system,** Christopher F. Ciliberto & Gertie F. Marx, World Federation of Societies of Anaesthesiologists, Issue 9 (1998) Article 2: Page 2 of 3, http://www.nda.ox.ac.uk/wfsa/html/u09/u09_004.htm (rib expansion and lung capacity)

Index

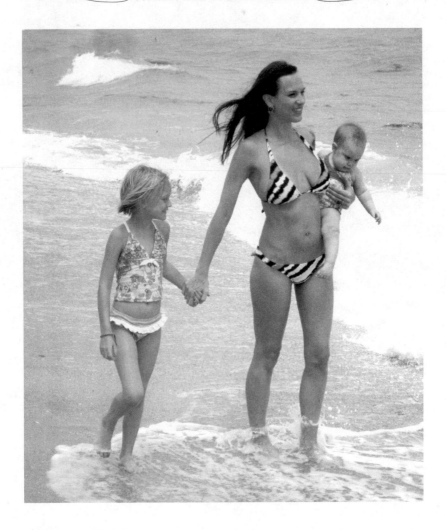

Peggy Emch has dedicated many years to the study of nutrition, with her main research interests being pregnancy, PCOS, food sensitivities, and the robust health of traditional peoples. After decades of suffering from various illnesses, she tried many different diets in attempt to heal herself, until she finally had success with simple, traditional foods.

Peggy is the blogger of the highly successful Paleo parenting website theprimalparent.com. As an author, speaker, and traditional foods advocate, she is proud to have changed the lives of countless children and adults with her guidance and counsel. Peggy graduated from the University of Colorado with a B.S. in mathematics and a B.A. in philosophy. She lives in Colorado with her simple-foods, Colombian husband and two well-nourished children.